EAT
SLEEP
TANTRUM
REPEAT

Also by Rebekah Diamond, MD

Parent Like a Pediatrician

EAT
SLEEP
TANTRUM
REPEAT

HOW TO PARENT LIKE A PEDIATRICIAN AND KEEP YOUR TODDLER HAPPY AND HEALTHY

Rebekah Diamond, MD

CITADEL PRESS
Kensington Publishing Corp.
www.kensingtonbooks.com

CITADEL PRESS BOOKS are published by

Kensington Publishing Corp.
900 Third Avenue
New York, NY 10022

PUBLISHER'S NOTE
This book is sold to readers with the understanding that while the publisher aims to inform, enlighten, and provide accurate general information regarding the subject matter covered, the publisher is not engaged in providing medical, psychological, financial, legal, or other professional services. If the reader needs or wants professional advice or assistance, the services of an appropriate professional should be sought. Case studies featured in this book are composites based on the author's years of practice and do not reflect the experiences of any individual person.

All Kensington titles, imprints, and distributed lines are available at special quantity discounts for bulk purchases for sales promotions, premiums, fund-raising, educational, or institutional use. Special book excerpts or customized printings can also be created to fit specific needs. For details, write or phone the office of the Kensington sales manager: Kensington Publishing Corp., 900 Third Avenue, New York, NY 10022, attn Sales Department; phone 1-800-221-2647.

CITADEL PRESS and the Citadel logo are Reg. U.S. Pat. & TM Off.

10 9 8 7 6 5 4 3 2 1

First Citadel trade paperback printing: October 2024

Printed in the United States of America

ISBN: 978-0-8065-4165-5

ISBN: 978-0-8065-4166-2 (e-book)

To P, B, and L, with all my love

Contents

CONTENTS

Contents

EAT
SLEEP
TANTRUM
REPEAT

Introduction

Hello and welcome from your friendly neighborhood pediatrician mom. Many of you will remember me from such hits as (1) *Parent Like a Pediatrician* take one (for your baby's first year), (2) social media–based guidance @parent likeapediatrician that helped keep you sane during the trials and tribulations of pandemic parenting, and (3) putting myself all over the internet to remind you that the secret to being an amazing parent has been inside you all along.

For those who are new here and may not be familiar with my stress-free, scientific, safe, and 100 percent pediatrician parent–approved approach to child-rearing, let's start with the basics. First things first, congratulations! You are doing amazing—surviving and even thriving during this incredible journey we call parenting. You made it through the first year (!!!), which is no small feat. It's actually a huge feat. The first months of parenting are easily one of the most overwhelming times of a human adult's life. And you came out of it intact, with a growing, blossoming child to show for it. What's more, you are still taking the time to seek out quality guidance for your ongoing journey. Congrats and well done, truly.

I'm delighted to say that you've found it—quality guidance, that is. This book is meticulously designed to keep you on track and to help you navigate the very different and very real challenges that the toddler years bring. And a comprehensive guide that covers each of these new challenges might be something you didn't even realize you needed. While there is an endless supply of books for parents of newborns (not all of the same quality, of course, and I hope *Parent Like a Pediatrician* has been helping you cut through the noise!), it seems like now you've been left mostly to your own devices. Sure, there are issue-specific niche books teaching you about common topics such as tantrums. There's also, as always, plenty of confusing, overwhelming online advice to sort through. But a comprehensive guide to tell you what to expect, what really matters, and how to handle the next few years in your parenting adventure? It doesn't seem to exist!

Until now. And not only does it exist, but I've also made sure it's something that truly makes your life easier. This book is your one-stop shop for toddlerhood, a time that is about so much more than any single challenge. Not just tantrums (don't worry, though, we'll tackle tantrums here too!) but a brave new world of sleep regressions, toilet training, vaccine appointments, outdoor play, picky eating, childhood sexuality (!), screen time battles, and more. As pediatrician visits become less frequent, these chapters will help fill in knowledge gaps that pediatricians (like me!) wish parents didn't have. And as you gain knowledge, you'll not only preemptively know what to expect, but you'll also be better prepared to troubleshoot issues as they arise—and know when to bring your pediatrician on board to help.

Because even though you've gained so much confidence, and are so much wiser, experienced, and more able to take on the challenges that lie ahead, there are always ways to make things easier. It's not the same newborn chaos you've just survived, but parenting a toddler is exhausting and *hard*. This book will lay it all out in one place, help you triage which topics need some of your still-precious attention and energy, and give strategies you can use to make things better—in your specific situation, according to your own unique parenting style.

I've curated a comprehensive list of toddler topics so you'll be maximally prepared. And, importantly, I'll present these chapters to you in a way that's maximally helpful. Forget those lists of "to-dos" and "to-don'ts," and forget essays full of inaccessible psychology that confuses more than it clarifies. This book keeps all the important science, laid out plainly, so that you know that there's reason underlying my balanced framework. Then it gives tangible guidance and key takeaways—truly helpful tips without stressful, prescriptive philosophies—showing you the range of safe, realistic options to choose from. In the end, you'll learn how to parent confidently, relying on your instinct (combined with some reputable information) to face each challenge that comes your way.

In the end, feeling empowered in your choices is the most important goal parents can set. While it should be an easy aim to achieve, the internet unfortunately continues to run fierce interference. You'll still find endless posts, stories, articles, texts, and blogs intent on convincing you that modern parenting is impossible. You'll find outrageous demands, insidious pseudoscience, and a whole lot of fearmongering. It's a nasty game designed to hook you on unnecessary advice, shill useless (and even harmful) products, and generally erode your well-earned confidence in the name of profit and power.

Never fear, I'm still here. Our society demands more and more of parents while giving us less and less. Instead of receiving the resources and common-sense guidance we need, we are told to stress over every tiny decision and even sacrifice our own sanity—without real good reason. In this overcomplicated day and age, it's all too easy to forget that parenting is meant to be a joyful experience! It should be, and it can be. This book (and my whole vibe, IRL and online) are all about restoring joy—by providing the information and assurance you need to make the best choices for your family. All the safety, all the science, none of the unnecessary angst.

Before we dive into the nitty-gritty and lay down some sweet guidance, it's time for a bit of brief housekeeping. The chapter topics may have changed, but the rules of the game are the same ones you've seen in my book and online platforms. First up is a reminder that my unique philosophy is grounded in equal parts science and common sense. I can't help but incorporate evidence and expertise into my work. As a board-certified pediatrician, my training includes four years of medical school, three years of pediatrics residency, plus continued daily work as a hospital pediatrician. And working as a hospital pediatrician means that sorting through data, staying up to date on health and safety recommendations for kids, and knowing how to translate scientific evidence into clinical advice is literally my job.

If you're worried that my background means I'm here to rehash American Academy of Pediatrics (AAP) handouts, evangelize rigid guidelines, or choose data over reason, there's no need to fret. It took me, tragically, way too long to realize just how unrealistic official advice can be, even when it's well-intentioned and based in science. Like so many pediatrician parents, having my own child completely changed how I practice medicine. I understand now that evidence and clinical insight matter only if they are translated into guidance that is realistic and reasonable enough to follow. It's why this book will again ditch strict guidelines and impractical, overwhelming advice that seems to be created in a vacuum, seemingly unaware of what it means to be a modern parent.

I'm also not afraid to be honest about the limitations behind official recommendations. My background means that I understand why AAP guidelines are great starting points, grounded in biology and whatever evidence we have available. It also means I know how the sausage is made and have a deeper understanding of what is really driving these rules and policies. Sometimes there's a lot of good data, and in these cases, I'll help you do your best to stick as closely to

by-the-book rules as possible. Other times, there's still a pau-
city of solid evidence behind our recommendations. I'll be
honest, happily sharing which hot-button parenting topics
are guided more by expert consensus and even guesswork.
We can embrace uncertainty, lean in to the wiggle room that
this gives us, while still making a scientifically sound assessment of risk and benefit.

An important caveat: understanding evidence and appre-
ciating science are complex tasks. It's tempting to think that
"data-driven" approaches are the only way to keep your parenting scientific. But these types of frameworks, which claim
to lay out all relevant studies side by side and let you choose
your own adventure, largely miss the mark. Real science is
about more than data, and pediatric medicine is about way
more than clinical studies. Even where we have rigorous trials
that inform our recommendations, breaking down the jar-
gon and helping you digest the research is just the first part of
my job. The hard work of evidence-based medicine is using
experience, clinical reasoning, and a big-picture understanding of science to decide if, when, and how research findings
can be applied to real life. The nuances of evidence-based
medicine mean that black-and-white parenting gospel, even
when it's backed by real science, never makes sense.

This book brings you the best of both worlds. You don't
have to ditch the scientific baby with the stressful, proverbial bathwater. We can skip the guilt, embrace the messiness
of parenting reality, all while *still* taking advantage of the
life-saving wonders of modern medicine. This means that

just like their "data-driven" counterparts, you can also forget about "guilt-free" approaches. Yes, I love a good #momfail meme, think "good enough" parenting is more than "good enough," and applaud movements that normalize parental imperfection. But "guilt-free" philosophies that abandon safe, commonsense guidance altogether are dangerous—and aren't the only way to restore your much-deserved confidence! You'll feel just as empowered (and raise a healthier, happier toddler) by using this book's framework. There is still no one "right" way to parent, but there are some safe and reasonable options that can guide decision-making. That's what I'm here to show you, and you'll see that, in many cases, rigid schedules and rules are less effective than sound philosophy that you can adapt to your own lifestyle. There's no need to choose between all-or-none official rules and "anything goes," free-for-all parenting. Instead, I'll help you create *your* own individual, sustainable, and scientific approach to child-rearing that works best for you and your family.

Because at the end of the day, who better than you to create your own personal parenting philosophy? You are the expert in your child, full stop. Parenting scripts, "try this, not that," advice, and any guidance you come across (even this book!) are only worthwhile if they *help* you feel empowered as a parent. It's great to seek expert advice and build up the tools in your toddler-taming arsenal. But ultimately, as cliché as it sounds, what you really need to reach your parenting potential has in fact been inside you all along.

Deep breaths. As we dive into the chaos of sorting myth versus fact and science versus pseudoscience, I promise you'll see that you are absolutely the best person to make decisions about your toddler's well-being. What seems like more work—making nuanced, personal choices based in a greater understanding of science and expertise—will quickly pay for itself, reaping rapid and remarkable rewards. You'll feel empowered in your innate ability to help your toddler reach their full potential, and even get permission to enjoy the experience! Yes, challenges are inevitable, but this book will teach you how to value your own health and happiness as much as you do your little one's—which, as luck will have it, benefits your child, too!

I'm also here to let you know that some things matter more than others. In life, we know there are plenty of times when the risks are unlikely to occur, but the consequences are bad enough to make preventive measures more than worthwhile (hello, seat belts and vaccines!). In a data-driven world, it's easy to get swept away in limited statistics and lose sight of the big picture. I'll help you triage the important *to-dos* and *to-don'ts* so you can agonize less and enjoy parenting more.

And I want to assure you that this book is for everyone. It's no secret that most mainstream, "comprehensive" parenting tomes have a very specific view of what the default "traditional" family looks like. But all families deserve to see themselves reflected in every corner of a comprehensive parenting guide. Universal guidance is only "universal" if it understands the challenges of those outside of the "traditional" parenting setup. My goal is to show you that you can be an amazing parent—even in face of the unique challenges presented by our society's disparities and inequalities—no matter what your family looks like.

At the end of each chapter, you'll see key takeaway points, which are here for you during those frantic moments when you need a quick refresher on what to do, or simply a reminder of why you are doing just fine (and don't need to waste precious minutes you could be sleeping going down a rabbit hole of parenting blogs!). These sections not only synthesize the most important information from each chapter but also give you a glimpse into the insights of my community of fellow pediatrician parents. My "5 out of 5 Pediatrician Parents Agree" seal of approval will let you know that pediatrician parents across the country echo and embrace my realistic, scientific, and compassionate advice.

This is the book I wish I had as a still-overwhelmed toddler mom. I desperately wanted to be told how to make safe choices for my child, and to be validated in the already safe choices I was making. It's time to take back parenting and enjoy it. No misinformation, no one-size-fits-all demands, no nonsense. Let's cut through the noise and keep things simple, without sacrificing any science or safety.

The internet is trying to break parenting. But we won't let it.

PART ONE

BEHAVIOR + DEVELOPMENT

CHAPTER 1

TIMERS, TOKENS, AND SYMBOLIC TOYS

Or How I Learned to Stop Worrying and Love My Toddler's Emotional Dysregulation

"**W**hy are toddlers monsters?"

I've heard—and to be honest, personally asked—some variation of this more times than I can count. The parents who pose this semi-rhetorical, semi-serious question love their kids as much as any Hallmark card would demand. But still, no amount of unconditional affection can take away the legitimate frustration of having your baby turn into a completely unruly, if still perfectly adorable, tantrum-prone beast.

The struggle is real, and in many ways unavoidable. Preparation is key. In this chapter, you'll learn what you can expect, how to set the groundwork for minimizing meltdowns, and how to manage your own emotional responses. Together, we can survive the behavioral storms that you'll navigate as your toddler learns to interact with their world and their own feelings.

It's impossible to choose just one story (or even two, or three) to illustrate how hard toddler behavioral management has been for me, my friends, and the parents I counsel. Should we talk about the time I gave my daughter the blue sippy cup instead of the orange one (how *could I* do that to her?)? In the blink of an eye, my new rug was covered in cranberry juice, and it took all I had to focus on my own breathing in my overstressed, sleep-deprived, and typically running-late-to-whatever-important-meeting-I-had state. Or how about when I cut the peanut butter sandwich in half when clearly it should have been served uncut? My two-year-old looked me dead in the eye, said, "I will *not* eat this one. I need a new sandwich now," then mashed it swiftly into a gooey bread ball and threw it with impressive athletic ability across the room.

In those moments, as a frazzled parent, I felt frustrated and defeated, but looking back now, it's hard not to laugh. It's no wonder the "why is my toddler mad at me?" TikToks are so popular. Toddlers can be irrational (to us, at least), unpredictable, and absurd. They also have the power to devastate us with their comments. Swapping toddler war stories is a rite of passage, as parents across the globe unite amid the challenges of how to deal with the most infuriating behavior imaginable—don't these kids know how hard we're working to make their lives as happy as possible?!—that comes from the creature we love more than anything in the entire world.

It's a universal, tragicomic mess. Understanding *why* this mysteriously monstrous behavior is happening is the first step to conquering it (or at least your reaction to it!).

Why Are Toddlers Monsters?

We've established that every parent on the planet deals with toddler meltdowns and other assorted behavioral outbursts, but *why* are all toddlers monsters?

Let's start with some basic science behind emotional processing specific to toddler development. Yes, much of this deeply challenging behavior is completely "normal." But even more important, most of it is also adaptive, fitting into a bigger picture of how little brains are learning to navigate and cope with the expanding, unpredictable world around them.

Research on toddler behavior focuses a lot on something called "self-regulation," which is a bucket term that refers to a group of skills your child is developing at this stage. When these skills are put together, they ultimately create a person's ability to guide goal-directed activity, especially when circumstances around them change over time. In plain terms, self-regulation is the anti-tantrum—a complex brain biochemical ballet that lets a person create a custom, careful response to the outside world based on the signals they receive. It's about taking emotions and combining them with cognitive processes so that reactions have meaning and serve a purpose.

There are a lot of neuronal networks involved in this very elaborate, rapidly developing decision-making dance. Managing emotions is a big one, as is something called "effortful control," where your brain suppresses a primary response that isn't appropriate in the circumstance and instead turns to a more acceptable action. Self-regulation also depends on being able to focus and shift attention, then being able to activate and inhibit specific behaviors. In short, it's complicated! Choosing the "right," or even less destructive, response to a stressor is a learned skill. And there's no toddler who can do this well, consistently. Heck, most adults are still working on this (or, at least, they should be!).

Getting from point A (an infant with extremely limited capacity for self-regulation who depends on caregivers for soothing in most situations) to point B (a preschooler with some basic self-regulation ability) is one of the biggest developmental milestones of toddlerhood. Around twelve to eighteen months, most toddlers gain the developmental ability for self-control, which marks the beginning of a rapid period of growth in self-regulatory skills. This means that toddlers' brains are working in overdrive, constantly creating and refining neural pathways based on the input they receive and how they process it.

To summarize: your one-year-old starts to rapidly develop some (still basic) brain connections that form the backbone of self-regulation. As these skills grow exponentially, we start to expect more of them, putting their newfound, primitive ability to make logical, emotionally challenging decisions to the test almost immediately. *Can you wait one minute until Mommy puts down her hot coffee before I fix that toy for you? I know you wanted the T. rex shirt but it's in the wash, I only see the pterodactyl one, can we put that one on?* The simplest requests require toddlers to exercise novel, rudimentary skills and suppress the urge to scream and cry—a response that just months ago was considered totally acceptable. It takes practice—in the form of meltdowns—for your little one's emerging abilities to strengthen and kick in. And all the while, your toddler is learning new self-regulatory skills by watching others—especially you—navigate tough choices, seeing that they, too, can start to make goal-directed decisions, even when they cause real emotional distress.

Whew, that's tough stuff. A lot of complicated feelings and science. Add in your toddler's limited language and communication abilities, and the fact that most of their daily activity is out of their control and often unpredictable, and it's no wonder that every minor discomfort or inconvenience they face seems to lead to an irrational sob. They're frustrated; they're learning; they're doing the best they can.

And so are you. Frustration is normal for both of you. The idea that you will respond to each situation perfectly and always know exactly what to say or do is just as illogical as your toddler's meltdown will be when you start to read their bedtime books in the "wrong" order. Just as we often expect toddler responses to be logical by our own standards, it seems that parenting guides are increasingly expecting *parent* responses to be perfect by some unproven, equally impossible standard. Let all that go and focus instead on being present, deliberate, and confident that you will find an approach to managing toddler behavior that works specifically for *you* and your child.

Without further ado, here are some of the guiding principles—and concrete strategies—that helped me get through the toddler years with minimal collateral damage.

The Pediatrician Mom's Guide to Low(er)-Stress Parenting: Toddler Dysregulation Edition

1. Set developmentally appropriate expectations.

Years of personal growth and therapy have taught me that expectations are everything. I owe a good chunk of my evolving happiness to the fact that I've learned to create more realistic goals and to better anticipate the fact that life will often not meet my desires. The phrase "lower your expectations" has blossomed from a dark joke to a liberating mantra.

It's the same for your child. Your child is incredible, adorable, wondrous, and capable of amazing things. Your child is also a child, and at this point a small, cognitively immature one. It's all too easy to focus on our responses to "bad behaviors," or plan how we will enforce any "rules'" we make. But I find that I can avoid a good amount of conflict altogether when I adjust my expectations. No, I'm not a fan of anything-goes parenting. It's great to have rules (and even consequences, which we'll talk about in our next chapter about tantrums). I'm just also here to let you know it's okay to triage. Would I have preferred that my daughter not put stickers on my walls during covid lockdown? Sure, but it didn't bother me that much, it wasn't hurting anyone, and I didn't have the bandwidth to enforce a no-sticker rule if I were to have made one. Throwing food on the floor annoyed me, but she was eighteen months old when this peaked. I was focused on social meals and adventurous eating, and I knew that altering this particular aspect of her mealtime "play" would be an uphill battle if I wanted to keep promoting food-exploratory behavior. Developmentally, it would have been challenging-to-impossible for my daughter to understand that messy investigation of the feel, taste, textures of the foods I offered her was encouraged; that pushing or even spitting up undesired morsels onto her high chair's tray was more than fine; but that tossing rejects onto the floor somehow crossed a line. With her early-toddler logic, language, and comprehension abilities, such a seemingly reasonable limit would have been arbitrary and needlessly frustrating for her. And even if I hadn't been worried about cleanliness getting in the way of culinary adventurousness, the bottom line was that I still had to triage. There were plenty of other behaviors that annoyed me far more—hitting, biting, wanton destruction of objects in my purse, for example—and required more thought and energy to discourage.

And the best part? You don't have to address every single "bad behavior" in real time to make sure it goes away. Waiting until your toddler is developmentally ready to follow a limit—especially if you're strategically focusing your limit setting on the other behaviors they *are* able to understand and that *you* have the bandwidth to enforce—won't cause irrevocable harm. Contrary to what some will still have you believe, you're raising a human, not training a dog. Parenting advice rooted in behavioral psychology—which is based largely in the assumption that all behaviors are the result of near-constant, cause-and-effect associations—are simplistic and inaccurate. We can embrace our ability to shape our child's behaviors while realizing just how much variability there is in the process. In the end, it's more about patterns than single interactions, meaning our kids are doing a *lot* more work than we give them credit for. Ultimately, their little brains are able to incorporate all types of input—trends in our limit setting, the behaviors we model, the thoughts and feelings we verbalize, the actions of their peers—in order to reach each behavioral milestone. By focusing on the big-picture patterns of what you do, you'll help your toddler reach their full potential—on their schedule, and without the extra stress.

In the end, perfect is the enemy of good. Before setting a limit, take a moment to decide if it's something you care about and if it's something your kid is even developmentally able to adhere to. As your little one battles near-constant psychological obstacles on the test that is toddler life, it's okay to grade on a curve.

2. Give them emotional tools in advance.

Building my family's emotional toolbox was one of the toddler tasks I enjoyed most. Yes, I'm a pediatrician with a basic background in psychology. It makes sense that I might take a shining to this topic more than most. But I think the main reason I found this aspect of behavioral management to be my favorite was that it was *positive* in the fullest sense of the word. It's always easier—for kids and adults alike—to add than subtract, to say yes instead of no, to feel like you are building instead of limiting. Working alongside your child to improve both your knowledge and expression of emotions can be an incredibly rewarding experience.

Laying the groundwork is simple. You can start just by naming emotions as you experience them, and helping your toddler do the same. When I told my husband about my day at the dinner table, my daughter heard examples of how I felt angry at whatever work drama had just presented itself. As we struggled to make it out of the house on time, I didn't shy away from expressing my frustration at the fact that searching for my daughter's stegosaurus sweater (no other outfit could possibly do) would undoubtedly make us late. I explained how I was sad when I personally lost something, missed a friend, or met my own personal daily disappointments. My daughter learned how I, too, got nervous about many of the activities I ultimately just had to do, building trust when it came time to face her own fears and making her "bravery" not about negating her anxiety but trying mommy-approved, safe activities despite them. I also made sure to name the positive feelings—joy, excitement, calm—I felt every day (especially when I was with her!). Extending this to others—asking other caretakers, family, and friends about their feelings and modeling an empathetic response—will take it to the next level. And there's an abundance of high-quality books, music, movies, and programs that are designed specifically for toddlers to identify and begin handling their very big feelings.

With time, you'll start to incorporate some higher-level emotional education. As you work on calling out big feelings, you can take the next step to validate them fully. When I described how enraged I was at my workplace conflict du jour, I gave myself verbal permission to feel that anger: "Wow, it really made me so mad when I couldn't get the patient the medicine they needed. It makes sense I had such a big feeling because I really care about that patient and really wanted them to have that treatment." The next pro step is to call out how—even though you yourself had such a big emotion, which made sense since people frequently get angry when things don't happen the way they think they should—your behavior was something you could still control. My daughter learned early on that all emotions were okay but certain expressions of them simply weren't. I may have wanted to scream, kick, or hit when the health-care system denied my patient appropriate care (I frequently have this urge), but I didn't. I could feel whatever I wanted to feel, I just couldn't choose violence. "I can be angry!" became my daughter's favorite catchphrase during meltdowns, with the implication that yes, she could feel whatever intense emotions came her way. But she still was responsible for managing the choices she made in expressing them. Separating feelings from actions is one of the biggest tasks that toddlers face (and most adults are still developing) as they strengthen their emotional regulation skills, a challenge we'll dive into more in our tantrum chapter. It's also a key part of developing your personalized framework to help replace hitting, biting, kicking, screaming with the more productive anger-management strategies (deep breathing, hugs, crying, punching pillows, throwing blankets) that we'll cover as well. Validating emotions doesn't mean anything goes, nor does it mean your toddler will have a carte blanche for id-fueled aggressive outbursts. Quite the opposite. Instead, embracing emotionally responsive, nurturing parenting is a crucial step to reducing the frequency and intensity of tantrum-fueled physical attacks.

3. Give choices.

When it comes to toddler behavior, nothing is a cure-all—and those "try this, not that" memes on social media often frustrate me more than they help. That being said, I was genuinely shocked to find that focusing on giving my daughter a limited number of choices—rather than just telling her what to do—seemed to avert nine out of ten meltdowns.

Your mileage will vary, and this may end up being less of a godsend and more of a helpful tool. Either way, it's worth trying. I found giving two to three choices to be the sweet spot, and I quickly began to give choices for almost every task of the day. Do you want to brush your teeth first or put on pajamas first? Do you want yellow or blue socks? Should we clean the macaroni and cheese off the floor with a paper towel or a cloth?

Get creative and incorporate giving this kind of controlled autonomy as it works best for you. Maybe you'll exceed your wildest dreams like I did one wintry morning. My two-year-old grabbed my hot coffee off the table and was ready to bolt with it across the living room. Instead of running or yelling, I somehow managed to keep my composure. I asked, "Do you want to hand that to Mommy yourself, or do you want me to come and grab it from you?" To my utter amazement, she stepped carefully toward me and surrendered the mug right over. Who says magic isn't real?

4. *Build your arsenal.*

Your toddler's world is even more out of control to them than it is to you. There's no way to regain complete control, but there are plenty of ways to be deliberate in your own choices. And there are also ways you can help provide some structure to your toddler's chaotic world so that things are just a little bit easier.

One of my favorite strategies is a visual schedule. This became a lifeline of ours during the pandemic, when the everyday lack of predictability all toddlers face turned into complete turmoil. Could we go to the playground today? Was Mommy going into the hospital to work? There were times when I genuinely didn't know the answer to basic questions like these until the night before. So when I found resources on making visual schedules online, I jumped on the opportunity. As the type of parent who finishes most of my daughter's crafts after she loses interest, making a custom-ized calendar with removable Velcro photos of my daughter engaging in different activities throughout the day was a fun assignment. But any basic visual schedule will do the trick, and the internet is filled with printouts and Pinspiration to meet your needs.

Quickly, setting up the next day's visual schedule became part of our nighttime routine. We mapped out the upcoming day, and when she woke up, we reviewed it again. It sat in our living room for her to reference as needed, and we even found ourselves making makeshift schedules on vacation. On extended family trips I became famous as the schedule maker, and more often than not it was the *toddlers* who came and asked *me* to sketch out the day with whatever crayons and scrap paper we could find. My initial surprise at the constant request soon made perfect sense; who wouldn't want to insert whatever amount of predictability they could into this increasingly uncertain world?

A few other personal favorite techniques that I often use work to create structure amid the chaos. While your toddler may not be *quite* as feral as the characters in *Lord of the Flies*, they may similarly benefit from a conch shell–esque, turn-taking symbol. It's something you'll likely notice in daycare or other group settings, be it an official object that kids pass back and forth to signify their turn, or the "sharing stegosaurus" I made up desperately during one playdate, a firm yet fair arbiter who told my daughter and her friend when it was time to pass on their toy to the other.

And, of course, no arsenal would be complete without a mention of the timer, a tool as beautiful as it is simple. I have yet to meet a parent who hasn't found some use of a timer to be helpful, which of course makes tons of sense. Toddlers are terrible at understanding time, and "two minutes" could be anywhere from three nanoseconds to three hours as far as they are concerned. How much your child wants, needs, or benefits from timers will depend on them, but it's a good bet there will be some real utility. Maybe it's just for transitions between routine activities, like when it's time to move from the swing set (Mommy's arms are tired!) to the slide during a playground trip, or when encouraging a calmer shift from enthusiastic pretend play to less exciting bath time. Turn taking is another prime example where countdowns can work wonders. A two-minute warning that comes with a disappearing orange circle and an iPhone Marimba alarm may be all you need for your toddler to peacefully relinquish that loud, new plaything they're hogging once their time is up. Or maybe your kid will request timers and even want to sit and watch them to calm and reset, something that absolutely does happen. Kids who struggle more with transitions—whether it's their temperament, related to an underlying behavioral diagnosis, or just a phase they're going through—benefit especially from external cues. But no matter your child's particular needs, timers, tokens, and symbolic toys, when used frequently, consistently, and together, give the structure all toddlers need to understand what transitional challenges lie ahead—an understanding that's paramount to preparing for, adapting to, and coping with these transitions.

5. Just you wait.

Patience isn't just a virtue, it's a lifesaver when it comes to toddler dysregulation. When in doubt, wait. Take a breath and don't respond. Did I mention, it's great to wait?

Seriously, taking a moment before responding is a great idea in life, and a staple of my own personal journey toward being a less reactive, more regulated human adult. There are many benefits, not least of all being able to cool yourself off and feel (even just slightly) more in control. It works wonders for toddlers, too. It helps them learn self-regulation by seeing how you don't immediately react. And it gives them a chance to respond to whatever is frustrating them on their own, practicing their own self-regulatory skills early on. I am still frequently surprised by how just taking five seconds before responding to pre-meltdown whines and demands (which feels like an eternity) gives my daughter the opportunity to engage in her own problem-solving, sometimes avoiding a full-blown meltdown altogether. Sure, she may have had a screaming fit that one time she *needed* the yellow truck—that she hadn't touched in six months—now that her playmate decided to take it off the shelf. But a scream was all that she needed. My five-second pause after her yelling was done was enough time for her to fix the problem herself, and simply move on to another toy.

6. Set safety limits.

It's more than okay to have a few nonnegotiables. Limits don't make you a less loving parent, something we will dive into in lots of fun, scientific detail later. I set a lot of safety limits, which has helped me be more flexible in situations where the threat of physical harm is less imminent. One example is stairway meltdowns. My daughter has learned that tantrums on the stairs are dangerous and absolutely not permitted, something I explained time and time again as her behavioral outbursts escalated, coincidentally, while on the stairway. If she didn't move herself to solid ground (which she, of course, never did for the first dozen or so attempts), I would lift her up and carry her to a safe location. Eventually, she was able to abide when I reminded her that "we cannot yell, hit, scream, or move unsafely on the stairs, ever, please come back downstairs now," if she wasn't too far along in the meltdown process. If not, or if the situation were too emergent for an attempted reminder (hello, sidewalk tantrums where toddlers crumple dangerously close to street traffic), I scooped her to safety immediately and didn't give it a second thought.

7. Stay positive.

There's lots of hype around different parenting styles, with "positive parenting" referring to specific strategies that we'll review in the tantrum chapter. I'm not here to espouse any rigid approach as a requirement. You'll decide which philosophy best meets your needs, if any. But in general, if you are looking for something to "do" in a specific situation, you'll find your best bet is choosing the "positive" option. In the broadest sense of the word, I'm a fan of "positive" parenting. Praise over punishment, hugs over scripted time-outs, or just shifting your own energy toward positive interactions. Instead of focusing too much of your own attention on the stress and mess, be present for the times when you and your toddler are enjoying each other and the world around you. A quick mental shift will help both of you appreciate just how much of your loving relationship is going right and just how well you both are doing overall as you navigate life's increasing challenges. This appreciation also acts as reinforcement for your toddler, making it more likely that they continue to choose the behaviors that bring everyone peace and joy—a win, win!

8. *Embrace natural consequences.*

In an attempt to minimize the use of traditional "punishment," it can be easy to feel like there's no way to teach cause and effect. But you can definitely find ways to add some basic "stakes" to your child's actions. Lots more to come on how all-or-none parenting philosophies miss the mark, and why incorporating rewards, time-outs, and more classic consequences may be something you choose to do. But even without these, you can plan on using natural consequences to your advantage.

Examples are endless, but here are a few good ones. When my daughter struggled to share, grabbed, hit, yelled, or otherwise was an unpleasant playmate, I told her the truth: I didn't want to play with her anymore, and neither would other kids. If this information didn't redirect behavior on its own (which it often didn't, especially not at first), I followed through—kissing my sweet two-year-old, telling her that I loved her and would play later once she calmed, then withdrawing my participation midgame. Sometimes I sat there and waited for her to regroup (or for the inevitable tantrum to erupt), sometimes I walked away and worked through my own frustration with our famous iPhone countdown timer and deep breathing. I felt calmer, she saw that her behavior had consequences, and I got to throw in a quick mindfulness-modeling session as an added bonus.

You'll quickly find that the opportunity to lean in to natural consequences are everywhere. Once I fully embraced this approach, it seemed that every situation could benefit from incorporating this type of cause-and-effect redirect, even if I had to get a little creative. My favorite example occurred one day when I was trying desperately to gently coax my daughter into helping me clean her disastrous array of toys that she had strewn in play across the living room. No amount of encouragement landed, and I realized our discussion had truly hit a wall when she told me, "I'm the boss of my own body, Mommy. You can't boss me around!"

I was proud to see that my lessons in bodily autonomy and the groundwork I was laying for consent had landed. And I was a little proud, I'll admit, that she had cleverly found a way to use my words against me. It was time to stretch beyond my usual semi-scripted responses.

"Yes," I replied, "that's true. You're the boss of your own body and you never have to do anything with your body that makes you uncomfortable, ever. No one can make you. You're in charge and make those choices. But there are still rules about what keeps everyone safe and choices that keep people safe and happy. You can choose not to clean up, but there are consequences. If we can't keep the living room clean, there won't be space for people to come over and play. And if we can't figure out how to put toys away, I won't have room for more toys in the future. So that's just something to think about."

I could see the wheels turning, as she contemplated the prospect of a life without the typical influx of playdates and presents. And wouldn't you know, just seconds later, my toddler grabbed my hand and brought me to the living room, demanding I join her in an immediate cleanup. It may not be every time, and it may not be right away. But toddlers absolutely understand cause-and-effect. When age-appropriate natural consequences that matter to them are at stake, they can play a powerful role in shaping behavior—minimizing meltdowns and even replacing more traditional types of "discipline" altogether.

9. Try fewer voices.

Consistency is key. As much as possible, all caregivers should operate by the same guidelines when it comes to interacting with your toddler. But putting up a united front, while super important, is just the first step. I found that next-level toddler dysregulation management requires a more nuanced look at how we are delivering our message, who was delivering it, and if everyone seems to be on the same page at the same time.

Don't stress or overthink it, and don't agonize over every interaction. We'll talk a lot in the next chapter about avoiding overly rigid scripts. No need to choreograph each line of dialogue or write a full screenplay. Just take a moment to observe and notice if there happen to be too many voices chiming in at once. I find things go best when there is one caretaker captain at a time, and when other caregivers who are around stay present and engaged (putting away your phone when you're not leading the toddler train is hard but extremely useful!). And when those little ones go loud, do your best to go quiet. Keeping a calm energy and maintaining focus can do a lot of heavy lifting when those big feelings lead to chaos.

10. Lean into pretend play.

One of the purest joys of toddler parenting is seeing their imagination blossom. It's truly incredible, and something you can totally take advantage of. In a good way, I promise!

Toddlers use pretend play every day, in more ways than is likely even visible to you. So lean in to it. This might mean simply paying attention to some of the themes of their pretend play and jumping in when the opportunity arises. There was a point where it seemed as if 99 percent of my parenting was directed at my daughter's imaginary friend, who allegedly was the one who was having a hard time controlling her anger, *not* my daughter. And if you don't have a pretend personification of your child's id to work with, you'll still find plenty of chances to work through feelings and behaviors using dolls, games, and general playtime conflict. Maybe you'll model some tough transitions with a favorite stuffed animal, or even engage your toddler in problem-solving when that stuffed animal "struggles" with their emotions. We did this constantly, to the point where I think every single toy in my daughter's room had a session "practicing" their bedtime routine and working through separation anxiety, as just one example.

Kids use imagination to explore their world, make sense of it, and sort through their very big feelings. Feel free to work through it with them! With one big caveat: you are *not* your child's play therapist. You are there to model behaviors, guide them through challenges, and above all else, have fun. You are not responsible for solo-tackling serious behavioral road bumps, and you do *not* need to turn joyful activities into psychoanalysis. In fact, you *should not* do this. Pay attention, be present, and incorporate play into life and vice versa. That's it!

11. Get silly.

When in doubt, make a fart joke.

I'm only (sort of) kidding. While I'm not a huge fan of potty humor, all toddlers, including my daughter, are. But regardless of what style of comedy your kid gravitates toward, humor can be a powerful tool. In addition to toilet jokes, our family relies heavily on absurdism. Maybe it was my decades-long love and appreciation of gonzo cinema that led me to rely on ridiculousness from an early age. My daughter was a willing participant, with a remarkable sense of humor that wouldn't let a near tantrum stop her from laughing at a good "bit." Your mileage may vary. But give it a try and you might be surprised. We use our toothbrush to brush our eyelashes, right? Pajama pants go on your arms, I'm sure of it! Your zany routine will likely garner laughs and will minimize meltdowns at least sometimes.

Why Why Why Why Why Why: Nurturing Inquisitiveness While Preserving Your Own Sanity

It's such a pleasure to watch your baby blossom into an inquisitive, curious, and critically thinking toddler. But even the most patient parent will ultimately reach a limit to how many times they can hear the word "why" without wanting to snap. Yes, it makes sense that there's so much "why" at this stage. Your toddler's language is growing rapidly, as are the cognitive processes that help them analyze the world around them. All of a sudden, they can *finally* ask questions about why things happen the way they do. When you think about it, it's amazing that the questioning isn't even more constant.

The nonstop interrogation is developmentally healthy and necessary. But it's exhausting. I remember some circular "why" conversations with my daughter that reached unimaginable levels of absurdity: *Why can't I use Mommy's hairbrush?* Because the bristles are too hard. *Why are the bristles hard?* Because Mommy has curly hair and needs that type of brush. *Why does Mommy have curly hair?* Because she was just born that way. *Why was Mommy born that way?* Because all people have different types and amounts of hair. *Why do people have different hair types?* Because their genetic code varies slightly enough to cause these differences. *Why does their genetic code vary?* Because of inheritance patterns, mutations, and meiosis, I think. *But why, why, why, why, why ... why? Mommy, why?*

Be kind to yourself. No human possesses the knowledge to satiate a toddler's inquiring mind, and even if they did, that's not the point. Your little one may keep asking questions until the end of time, no matter how thorough an explanation you've provided. So do your best, and if you get frustrated, you're in very good company. Pause, regroup, and do what it takes to keep your wits about you. Maybe you'll collect a few stock phrases to respond with; "I'm not sure, what an interesting question." Or maybe you'll just need to say, "I hear you," and wait until the interrogation reaches a natural lull.

Here are four other strategies I have found helpful:

1. **Give *yourself* choices.** As "why" interrogations escalated, I introduced a rule: I am allowed to say, "I don't know," and this is a response she has had to learn to accept. People don't know everything! But, if that wasn't satisfying (surprise surprise, it almost never was), she could respond, "Use your imagination." This meant I was allowed to tell a story instead. On one walk, unable to satisfy questions about who lived in a house down the road, I entertained myself by creating a long, complex backstory for the pretend families who had lived there over the decades. It passed

the time and was certainly more fun than walking home to the soundtrack of "Whyyyyyyyyyy?" wails echoing in the wind.

2. **Find other ways to entertain yourself.** I'm a self-proclaimed nerd, and being a doctor means that I have some basic scientific background. So I made a game of trying to remember as much physics, chemistry, and biology when answering the seemingly impossible. No, I don't think my daughter understood my description of cellular apoptosis as part of the answer to a series of questions beginning with "Why do fingernails grow?" But I sure had a good time flexing my premed biochem knowledge!

3. **Flip the script.** I became a huge fan of answering questions with questions. To encourage curiosity, I segued into related topics: "I don't know why cats make a 'meow' sound, but I do know a bit about how human voices work. Do you want to learn about that?" Sometimes, if she'd allow it, I'd ask her to guess or explain answers herself, trying to work through it with her. Why did *she* think snakes don't have feet? Was there a different way that they moved instead? This technique requires more time and effort, but if you have the energy, it can be an enjoyable way to analyze the world together.

4. **Take a page from medical rounds.** When I work with students and residents, I always give 100 percent

full credit if they answer, "I don't know, but I will look it up and report back." With a world of knowledge literally at our fingertips, it's hard to justify guessing when we don't have to. Foster investigation and finding sources from an early age; ask Siri, Google, Alexa, or any source of knowledge that is likely to have the answer. Heck, maybe you'll even go to the library and read a whole book about the earth's atmosphere when your explanation of why the sky is blue just doesn't cut it. It's a great opportunity to practice critical thinking and scientific literacy when looking for information.

THE BOTTOM LINE

5 out of 5 Pediatrician Parents Agree

1. Toddlers are behavioral monsters. Their emotional dysregulation is a rite of passage, as adaptive as it is normal. It's a critical part of your child's development.
2. There's no way to prevent all meltdowns or make the experience of dealing with an irrational tiny human completely stress-free.
3. There are, however, ways to improve the experience for both you and your child. Key strategies include setting developmentally appropriate expectations, modeling emotional regulation, focusing on your own reactions, pushing yourself to be patient, using tools that help your toddler feel more in control of their routine, embracing natural consequences, and leaning into humor and pretend play.
4. "Why?" questions are developmentally important but truly annoying. You can engage with them as much as your energy allows. Sometimes just listening or promising to look up information later, however, is all you'll have the bandwidth to do.
5. Your frustration with toddler irrationality does not make you any less of a loving parent.
6. When behavioral management goes "wrong," replace the guilt with reflection. Challenges and perceived missteps aren't failures, they're simply an opportunity to regroup and see if a different strategy makes more sense in your situation.

CHAPTER 2

TIME'S UP FOR TIME-OUT

Love + Limits + Patience – Rigid Parenting Philosophies = Your Ticket to the Lowest-Stress Tantrum Experience Possible

There's nothing more frustrating than the most unreasonable toddler behavioral meltdown, spurred by the most ridiculous trigger, which always seems to come *just* when you finally feel like you're getting the hang of this whole parenting thing. Tantrums may be normal, but they are always exhausting and frequently overwhelming—even for the most confident parents among us. In this chapter, I'll show you how centuries of research in behavioral psychology and resilience training, combined with a loving, empathic approach, create a winning framework for dealing with your toddler's hitting, kicking, screaming, throwing, and everyday meltdowns.

Toddler tantrums have always been a special rite of passage for parents and the little creatures they are trying to raise.

As a pediatrician, seasoned babysitter/auntie, and general fan of small children, I felt well prepared as my daughter entered her toddler years. Having spent most of my life around little kids, I entered this stage of parenting knowing that completely irrational emotional outbursts were the norm, not the exception. My expectations were realistic, and I reviewed enough resources (and gave myself enough preemptive pep talks) to set myself up for success. I knew patience was the name of the game, and I felt as primed as possible.

Around age one, the mini tantrums made their introduction into our daily routine. It was pretty much what I expected. Serving milk in a pink sippy cup instead of the blue 360-degree toddler cup? *How* dare *you, Mom!* I should have known better. And the deeply disproportionate outrage was kind of funny. I would just take a deep breath, try again, and file that one away for tantrum-meme material and cocktail-party parenting war stories.

But my confident calm was quickly eroded by circumstances—both typical and unprecedented. Around my daughter's second birthday, I noted a predictable uptick in outbursts. Work was busy, and we were completing a move to a new home. We were staying in the same neighborhood, but still, it was an upheaval for all of us. Emotions were high all around. We handled it all relatively well, and I made mental notes to spend a little more time building my tantrum arsenal when life settled down.

A few months later, things settled just as I hoped, and I had the time, energy, and psychological reserve to create a toddler behavioral plan that made the upcoming years a breeze.

Just kidding. A few months later was March 2020. I still haven't fully unpacked the trauma of being a hospital physician in our country's original COVID-19 epicenter. My family, like most of the country, was thrust into a completely new, terrifying, chaotic, dynamic, and entirely overwhelming way of life. I still feel lucky beyond measure to have come out with my health—and that of my friends and family—intact, a blessing of which more than a million Americans have been deprived. The losses are enormous and indescribable. I will always keep this in perspective when I look back on my own trials and tribulations, and when I reflect on the choices parents like myself have been forced to make over the subsequent years.

The unique challenges of pandemic parenting meant that a "normal," age-appropriate escalation in tantrum behavior was just the beginning. Kids are resilient, and my daughter navigated spring of 2020 —which turned into years of lockdowns, quarantines, closings, openings, reclosings, masks, distancing, and more—with inspiring perseverance. But this doesn't mean that it was easy for her, and it doesn't mean that it wasn't even harder for her parents. Tantrums escalated, were more frequent, grew more challenging, and were often triggered by whatever sudden routine change du jour we encountered.

We did the best we could. There were plenty of days where tantrums happened more than once (which, it turns out, can be normal even in non-pandemic times). But some days were better, and as time went on, I felt increasingly confident in the approach I created. I reviewed the expert guidance, brushed up on my pediatric behavioral psychology research, and developed a framework that ultimately empowered me to firmly but flexibly be the responsible, nurturing parent I always wanted to be. Not perfect, but perfect for my daughter, and trying above all else to give myself grace as new challenges continued to arise.

I'm here to help you similarly create your own unique, stress-reducing tantrum playbook. Tackling tantrum management could be a whole book in and of itself (in fact, there are tons of books out there that are entirely devoted to this topic, and you'll find my favorites linked on my website). But before you draw up a battle plan, it's always important to take stock and get a lay of the land. And while toddler meltdowns aren't technically war, it's barely an overstatement to say that they can certainly feel that way. Love is a battlefield, making big-picture strategy just as important as any in-the-moment coping techniques.

The Big Picture: Important Ground Rules as You Dive Into Tips, Tricks, Research, and Advice

1. Your child didn't read the textbook.

Your child is a person. I know you haven't forgotten this, but as you're inundated with one-size-fits-all parenting "hacks," it's natural to interpret normal deviation as something that's "wrong" with your child. This can even lead to guilt and self-blame; I see countless parents incorrectly internalize their child's behavioral idiosyncrasies or nonstandard response to typical behavior management strategies as signs of parental failure. They aren't. In medicine, we love to say that a patient "didn't read the textbook" when diagnosing conditions that don't meet strict diagnostic criteria. The truth is that perfectly "textbook" cases are the rare ones. It's what makes the art of medicine so challenging (and important). And it's the same for your family. Norms are norms, averages are averages, trends are trends. Your child, on the other hand, is your child. Only you and your kid are experts in their quirks, wants, and needs. This means that only *you* are the best judge of which strategies make sense. No one else, not even the experts. Nope, not even me!

2. *Patterns are what matters.*

By now we've firmly established that perfection in parenting is a lie. But even if we were to find some sort of mystical forest in which magical creatures called the Perfect Parent spend their fictional days, this fact would remain: You will have "off" days. I repeat, you *will* have off days. It may be a one-off, Alexander-style no-good, very-bad day, or it may be a full-on Lemony Snicket week consisting of a series of unfortunate events. Either way, it's okay.

Whether it's your kid's behavior, life's circumstances, or even your own response that's got you down, do your best not to catastrophize. We learn from our mistakes and need to teach our kids this is a good thing to do, too! Our actions matter, but they matter most in aggregate. Meaning, it's really the patterns of behaviors, the environment we create for our children, and our ongoing, evolving relationship with them that ultimately shapes their psyche. Use a bribe? Appease a public tantrum with unlimited screen time just to make it through? Maybe you even—*gasp*—lost your cool when your three-year-old smacked you in the face mid-meltdown? It will likely happen. And it won't be irrevocable, and it won't make you a failure. Take time, regroup, reflect. Your kid will be okay, and so will you. There's room to grow if you give yourself grace.

3. It's always okay to get personalized, expert help.

For real. No matter how "small" a challenge may seem to you, or how "simple" a question might feel, seeking expert guidance is an amazing option. Helping you with challenges is why experts exist! Individualized guidance from a pediatrician, psychologist, or certified expert in childhood behavior is a sign of strength, not failure. Yes, much of the variation we find in how kids act day to day and respond to parenting techniques is just that—variation. But sometimes it's a sign of other developmental issues that professionals are trained to recognize and treat. And many times, there's nothing but a strong-willed child, a challenging circumstance, or some other, nonmedical reason that your kid might be having a particularly hard time. Either way, phoning a highly trained "friend" is a great way to get extra support and individualized guidance.

4.   Any approach that is black-and-white is not the answer.

In the throes of lockdown and in-home meltdowns, I spent hours scouring social media for any potentially helpful script that would give me the perfect words to deal with my daughter's increasingly frequent outbursts. Over the course of months, I spent hours trying out different options and carefully modifying useful phrases to meet my needs and style. I rewrote, refined, or entirely threw out countless scripts. Ultimately I wound up with an evolving but generally stable catchphrase cache that I leaned on when high-riding emotions made it hard to think of verbal responses on the fly.

I like a lot of tantrum scripts, and I'm a big fan of memorizing some responses for when things heat up. I'll even share some of my favorites in the frontline strategies section later in this chapter. But scripts are tools, and tools are only valuable if they're helpful. If expert guidance starts to make you feel bad about yourself, is impossible to follow, or just isn't working for you or your kid, it's not the right guide for you. This may mean it's time to try a different approach altogether, but it may be as simple as adding in some line edits and ad libs. I always try to "perform" my parenting scripts with as much flexibility as possible. Sure, it's helpful to have some lines to recite, but obsessing over word choice and banning improvisation doesn't make a lot of sense. Split the difference and aim for a performance that lands somewhere in between the fully unscripted work of Larry David and the by-the-book plays of David Mamet.

While we're on the subject of "parenting scripts," it might be a good time for a tangent on "parenting philosophies."

A common question I get when discussing the world of parenting advice—from experts and parents alike—is about my own parenting philosophy. What "style" do I, Dr. Diamond, personally ascribe to? At first, the question confused me—what even is a parenting philosophy? As I became a parenting expert, I understood that this question was asking me to categorize myself as a follower of one of a handful of popular, modern, child-rearing approaches that I've become familiar with over the years (and which we'll break down in detail in the next section). I also learned that my answer is complicated: I like aspects of a variety of different expert guides but don't feel that any single title encompasses how I personally parent, or how I empower others to do so. On the one hand, I appreciate so many of these guides, and I've seen how they create frameworks, break down basic psychological concepts, and help parents become more mindful. On the other, it can be hard to separate "philosophies" from "brands" and keep the for-profit, black-and-white advice from undermining your parental confidence.

In the end, the real experts in tantrums understand that scripts are made to be modified, and that any overly rigid approach is a recipe for disaster. Remember, even for those beloved, groundbreaking pioneers like Spock and Ferber, there will never be a single voice that can perfectly dictate all your parenting choices—except your own. (Still not even me!)

The guides I use personally and professionally are the less-famous ones who piece together the evidence, give you a framework for what you might want to do, and help you find the style that works for you. (Sound familiar? I hope so, this is my biggest goal!) Remember: Any approach that's too rigid and doesn't allow for parents to be human is something to take with a grain of salt. That being said, some parenting philosophies are famous for a reason—and largely a good reason! They represent a shift from some of the more frustrating, widely held misconceptions about parenting and open the door to an individualized, lower-stress approach.

These days, the trend, generally speaking, is a pivot away from traditional, behavior-focused philosophy toward more emotionally attuned parenting strategies. There is in fact science supporting this transition, and I truly am happy to see so much thought put into the overall emotional well-being of children—and what we as parents can do to support it. But there isn't any single approach that boasts peer-reviewed evidence worthy of crowning it the winner of the Parenting Philosophy Olympics. The science we have is based on our growing understanding of child psychology—which informs the behavioral tips I've given so far—and data that deal more with broad strokes and the bigger picture. For example, a

2019 meta-analysis (the gold standard of academic review) collected available data on the relationship between various parenting practices and positive outcomes in children, like self-regulation (which we talked about in chapter 1). This review found that using positive strategies instead of negative (e.g., coercive behaviors and punishment) was associated with better child self-regulation. The highest levels of self-regulation among traditional parenting approaches were seen from those with both high levels of love and responsiveness and limit setting—a hallmark of what has been dubbed "authoritative" parenting. This improved self-regulation was long-lasting and linked to better self-regulation later in life. Other cited studies found a link between parents who modeled their own self-regulation and the ability of their children to self-regulate. Add this to decades of research on child development, the biology of attachment, and yes, some old-fashioned behavioral psychology, and a guiding principle emerges: kids need love, affection, guidance, and emotional modeling to thrive. Neglect has been off the table for ages, and traditional punishment is unnecessary and can be harmful.

So what does this mean for the different but similar, "unique" but overlapping, parenting styles you'll undoubtedly find online? Let's review some of the popular, trending parenting philosophies and the principles behind them to find out!

The Big, Wide World of Conscious Parenting, Gentle Parenting, Mindful Parenting, Intentional Parenting, Respectful Parenting, Unconditional Parenting, and Positive Parenting

As you scroll through your social media feed, you'll undoubtedly come across tips, tricks, and scripts adhering to one of these specific philosophies. We'll go into which aspects of these modern approaches seem to work best (and which caveats to keep front and center when taking any of this advice). If you're already confident that an individualized, philosophy-free approach is the way to go, feel free to jump ahead to the upcoming "frontline strategies" section where we put the best parts of these philosophies into action. I promise I won't be offended if you skim over or completely skip this deep dive into today's predominant parenting philosophies. Sometimes nitty-gritty breakdowns—that ultimately show you what not to do rather than what to do—add more noise and stress than they're worth. But I'm including this here because for many parents (myself included), a more in-depth look into what is really behind all those online trends can actually be helpful. I find it easier to embrace my own parenting style—borrowing from others when it makes sense, ignoring advice when it doesn't—once I understand the science and history underlying the guidance that's out there.

Still with me? Great. I wanted to start this section by creating a super scientific, organized taxonomy of the major modern parenting philosophies. The hope was to outline exactly what made each one unique, give you charts, Venn diagrams, tables, and all sorts of sexy schematics to cleanly delineate the boundaries of each official parenting philosophy.

But I failed. I'm not even trying to be glib; this really turned out to be an impossible task. It just isn't possible to definitively tease apart "gentle," from "mindful," from "conscious" approaches because they are so interconnected and rely on such similar founding assumptions and techniques. Sure, there are nuances in style, shifts in strategy, and subtle differences among them. I would never try to detract from the decades of work parenting psychologists have poured into these philosophies and the resources they create. But we can give credit where it's due and appreciate the work of experts without getting lost in academic discussion. I ditched taxonomies and instead am bringing you the big picture. What matters is principles, so let's break down the major ones you'll find in many (if not all) of these approaches.

1. Be mindful.

Universal to modern, emotionally attuned approaches is a focus on mindfulness. I totally dig it, as I hope you could guess from my favorite toddler dysregulation management strategies in chapter 1. Reflecting on yourself, understanding and untangling the relationship between big feelings and behavior, is an evidence-based way to help your child improve their own self-regulation. And, of course, there's more than a century of evidence bestowing the benefits of having a loving, attentive parent who responds with consistent affection, a common theme in all these approaches.

2. *Avoid punishment.*

Another uniting principle of trending parenting philosophies is pivoting away from punishment. It's something I'm also into, especially ditching harsh punishment and shifting toward natural consequences and/or positive reinforcement in their stead when behavioral shaping is needed. Head back to our first chapter to remind yourself that you are already doing a great job focusing on reinforcement and consequences over punishment. And while you're there, take time to review the other behavior-management strategies that you may or may not have already incorporated into your routine. Those mindfulness strategies really do work, over time, to decrease the number of undesired behaviors and outbursts. When all these strategies are put together, it's likely that the need for traditional punishment will be less apparent, making a primarily "positive" approach much more feasible.

Mindfulness does a lot of heavy lifting, and generally staying "positive" is a winning strategy. But tantrums happen, and they're not your fault. What we do as a parent matters a lot—in aggregate, especially—but your child is their own person. There is no single philosophy that will work perfectly for every child, and even the best, most tailor-made approach will fail to fully regulate your toddler. It's not developmentally possible! Your one-, two-, or three-year-old still has those immature neuronal connections that make advanced self-regulation as unnatural as it is unrealistic.

In short: there *will* be tantrums. How on earth will you deal with them? Does this mean that so-called unnatural consequences are canceled? Is time really *up* for timeout? Of course not. I personally found that replacing official time-outs with other strategies worked better for us, and I'll highlight my favorite tantrum tips and tricks in the next section. But a lot of my time-out–free parenting is mostly semantic—our use of a timer and meditation is what many would call a "time-in" or "reset." It's something your child's daycare or school will likely use if they don't still hold on to standard "time-out" practices. Which, it turns out, is totally fine. A fun fact that anti–time-out evangelists forget to mention? There's no evidence that time-outs, when used as part of a loving, thoughtful arsenal of parenting strategies, cause any actual harm.

3. Take it a step further and ditch rewards, too.

Some modern styles replace punishment with reinforcement—such as positive parenting, which likes positive reinforcement (rewards) just fine. But others—some forms of conscious, gentle, mindful parenting, for example—make it seem that stickers, treats, and even praise are legitimately harmful.

As always, it's a much more nuanced conversation than a simple ban on any behavior. The psychological principle behind this anti-reward approach is that your relationship with your child is an unconditional, bidirectional, dynamic one. This is true. But the next presumption—that using any behavioral modification strategy serves as a "manipulation" that undermines that relationship—is a real stretch. It's something I struggled with, finding myself needlessly stressed when social media posts made me feel as if using sticker charts and telling my daughter how smart she was made me a bad parent. Ultimately I realized that my loving, unconditional connection to my child is anything but "transactional," and that I can ignore anything that makes me feel less than thrilled with the relationship I am cultivating for us.

I see why anti-reward advocates push against primarily behavior-based parenting. When I talk about behavior-based science, old-school behavioral psychology, or behaviorists, I'm referring to approaches grounded in the premise that nearly all human actions are the result of preceding stimuli. When it comes to parenting, this usually leads to the assertion that the best way to shape behavior is through reinforcement and punishment. I'm a fan of calling out purely behaviorist strategies—like the very outdated rules equating toddlers with trained animals and mandating cry it out to sleep and three-day toilet training. It's actually an old clapback, with Dr. Spock and his acolytes similarly raging against strict behavioral psychology in the parenting space. But sticker charts, incentives, and other rewards are all very reasonable to keep in your toolbox. They're strategies that I have used and will continue to use, and you'll see them throughout the book when we talk about topics like toilet training and sleep training. And definitely, definitely, *definitely* ditch any extreme approaches that go beyond the limits of logic. There are ways to make praise constructive, be mindful of what we are reinforcing and how, and choose our words carefully. Saying that "praise is manipulative" or pretending "good job" is a bad word, however, ain't it.

It took me longer than I wish it had to fully realize this, and firmly ignore all guidance that tried to make me feel bad for *my* version of positive parenting. Plenty of sources strongly suggested that when I shouted "Great job!" after my two-year-old did a not-even-good-job-but-I'm-so-happy-she-tried job cleaning up her mess, I had caused some sort of nebulous long-term harm. That's nonsense. I love looking at patterns, being mindful, and the sociolinguist in me will always be down to see how we can optimize language to improve impact. But ditch any scripts that are based in shaky science—or any biological plausibility—and remember that the words that let you communicate lovingly and confidently with your child are the right ones.

4. Focus on your own responses, not your kid's.

The sometimes singular focus on a parent's *own* emotional response is commonly seen in parenting brands that use the "conscious," "gentle," or "mindful" label. As a prime example, the hallmark of traditional "conscious" parenting, an approach spearheaded by the very popular book *The Conscious Parent* by Dr. Shefali Tsabary, is encouraging parents to focus on their own responses and behaviors in order to be more thoughtful in responding to their children. This is founded on the premise that our own experiences, namely those from childhood, can shape how we view the world and inform what we decide is acceptable or not. By tuning into our own triggers, we can use our past to better, less reactively respond to our children's challenging behaviors. The hope is to be able to prevent negative patterns from perpetuating themselves, which starts by being mindful of our own reactions and internalized beliefs as parents.

It's not all-or-none, and it's not always-or-never. Understanding your own emotional and behavioral reactions when you can is great! My therapist will confirm that I've been working on my own reactivity, with a main goal of being the best parent I can be, for years. Nonetheless, the constant reminder to emotionally separate myself from my daughter—an admirable goal I was already working on—became, ironically, an emotional trigger.

Once, after a particularly stressful day of parenting, my social media scrolling brought yet another "say this, not that" video from an online tantrum guru. It felt like the expert was speaking directly at me when she explained how wrong it was to say "When you scream in my face, it makes me feel sad." Just five minutes ago, when my daughter had indeed screamed in my face for some inexplicable three-year-old reason, I had said those exact words to her.

It was a classic "mom fail." The guilt was automatic, visceral, and I felt a knot in my chest. I immediately went from feeling proud that I had calmly expressed my feelings and maybe even promoted empathy—no small feat when you're exhausted, have a migraine coming on, and a three-year-old's tantrum unleashes all its fury aimed at you—to feeling like an awful parent. According to the online expert, I should have explored my daughter's feelings in real time, acknowledging that she must have felt really upset to react like that. Looking back, I understand why I cried in discouragement. But I soon realized that there wasn't anything so "terrible" about my calm reaction—one that I had been using successfully and confidently for over a year. There's no evidence that linking a child's behavior to someone else's feelings is inherently harmful. And even if there were, scripts always need to be modified. Context, timing, and each individual situation all trump data. I resolved to be more judicious in how much I internalized the strategies that came my way. Even from sources and philosophies I otherwise found useful.

A parenting philosophy should fit your parenting style, not the other way around. Studies show that self-efficacy (confidence in your ability to raise your child) has long-term benefits for your child. There's no specific script or sole source of guidance that can replace the benefit of how you feel empowered in your parenting techniques. And even if a single script had data behind it, I still wouldn't recommend rigid adherence. We don't even do this in health care! The art of medicine is using those peer-reviewed studies in a way that makes sense for *your* patient. I've said it once and I'll say it again: just like my patient was not in the randomized controlled trial that recommended this treatment, your child was not in the test group for whatever guidebook you're using. Take what you need and leave the rest.

Now that we're on the same page about the benefits (and limits) of a tantrum guide, it's time to share mine. Think big picture and broad principles rather than the intricate details of any specific tantrum. Be as flexible as possible, and as kind to yourself as you can. What works in some instances won't work in others, with transitions and new environments being especially challenging and requiring on-the-fly adaptation.

And remember, getting through the tantrum era is exhausting! Treat yourself with as much grace as you would want your child to receive. It's not just what you need to get through it, but it's also crucial to creating a loving, open, and forgiving household environment—the key ingredients to nurturing emotional intelligence.

In the Weeds: Frontline Strategies to Get You Started as Tantrums Come Your Way

It's easy for me to preach nuance, tell you to ditch parenting scripts and follow your instincts. But you know what isn't easy? Dealing with a tantrum. I've been there, countless times. Having some basic tools and even favorite stock phrases is more than fine. You can stay flexible but also be prepared. And above all else, remember that the "when" is as important as the "what" or "how." Meaning, how you dive into a full-blown monsoon of a meltdown will be much different from your approach to a mini tantrum as it starts to ramp up.

I. During the calm (building a foundation and learning from past tantrums)

Take a moment to review the strategies in chapter 1 and remember that you have already set a strong foundation in emotional regulation. It's not just about preventing tantrums—although that is a very real perk. The frequent meltdowns you're seeing are undoubtedly less frequent than they would be if you hadn't already been so intentional in your parenting! And the tantrums that do come your way are easier for both you and your child to get through, even if you can't always see it, than they would be if you hadn't laid such a great emotional foundation.

II. As things ramp up (a.k.a. "escalation nation")

In the early stages of a tantrum—and sometimes in the middle, like an eye of the storm—you'll have periods where your child is only mildly melting down. It's not a period of complete calm, but it's distinct from the upcoming peak of the tantrum, where total dysregulation (those heaving sobs, uncontrollable screams, and violent rage) takes over. During this relatively calmer time, I found I could do some *very light* intervention. This isn't the same as what we worked on in chapter 1, which are strategies to use when your child has the emotional reserve necessary to engage in more challenging goal-directed behavior. Your expectations will be different; the aim here isn't to teach emotional processing or shape any behaviors in the longer term. Instead, your mission is simply to make it to the other side of *this* specific tantrum.

Here are some tools that helped me engage more productively with my daughter during the lulls and crescendos of her tantrum journey. You may find that they work incredibly well, not at all, only occasionally, or a lot more frequently than you thought. You know the drill: try them out, adapt based on the responses you're seeing, and incorporate them into your arsenal however best works for you.

1. Use humor.

Humor is one of the most versatile tools of parenting, and I say this not just because of my own personal love of comedy. I've found that it's one of the few tools that can work both when kids are pre-tantrum and when tantrums are already underway. My daughter could break mid-meltdown, especially during the upswing, to laugh at a particularly good joke.

2. Keep it quiet.

It's easy to meet yelling with yelling. Honestly, a big part of emotional escalation during tantrums is just the volume.

Any readers who come from a family that's loud like mine can recognize that multiple overlapping voices, often competing to be heard, quickly heightens the tension in any situation. So I try to meet screams with whispers as much as possible—at least when I am actually trying to be listened to. During a tantrum, your toddler's ability to process what you say is very limited. Just because you're loud and have been technically "heard" doesn't mean you've been listened to. I found that when I spoke quietly, and she had to pay attention to really hear me, she was more likely to actually take in what I was saying.

Does this mean that every time I begin whispering brilliant words of wisdom my child stops screaming and tunes right in? Of course not. And if it does work, it's rarely on the first attempt. I often give a quick invitation in a louder voice—"I see you're upset, let me know when you're ready to talk"—and check back in asking if she is ready until she, usually, eventually, comes over to engage.

3. Remind them of their choices.

You've already laid the groundwork for how to separate feelings from behavior. And you've already given lots of choices in how to manage feelings. Maybe you offer that timer you usually use to help with transitions, but now, instead of waiting for it to signal the end of someone's turn, you sit and watch it together. For us, this was more of a godsend than I could have ever anticipated. During almost every tantrum my daughter chose the anger-management strategy of "watching the orange go by." When she asked for this, I sat her on my lap and turned on my always-ready two-minute iPhone timer, and we breathed together as we watched the orange countdown tick away.

Having learned to proudly state, "I can be angry!" from an early age, we've also worked to pair this totally acceptable emotion with some totally acceptable responses. Throwing a blanket or pillow is a good one. We had already learned some mindfulness techniques, primarily because it was something I was learning for myself! When feelings and behaviors escalate, deep breaths are always encouraged, sometimes with that infamous timer and sometimes with other visualization tools. A favorite strategy I created during a fit of desperate inspiration was the "angry ball." During the worst of the tantrum years, we practiced breathing into an imaginary "angry ball" shaped by mommy's fingers that grew bigger with each breath and eventually blew away. Of course, hugs were *always* an option and are still one of the first things I offer when I see my daughter start to get upset. As a childless pediatrician, completely lacking insight into how behaviorism had snuck into my guidance, I painfully remember telling parents that hugs somehow "reinforced" the "bad behavior" of tantrums. I now know better, and hope that you feel empowered to physically comfort your child whenever and however you both need.

4. *Consider a reset or change in course.*

If things are ramping up, feel free to abort the mission. Meaning, maybe this activity or situation is just too stimulating. Maybe the fight isn't worth it and you change your mind. I used to think that revising a limit was the same as "giving in" to a "bad" behavior, but I have learned from the real experts that it's always okay to reassess. It's not all or none. I wouldn't suggest handing over that lollipop just because your three-year-old starts screaming in your ear, but I've certainly altered our plans when emotions were too high for everyone. For instance, one day at 7:00 p.m., already behind schedule for bedtime, the battle to bathe my pretty-clean toddler just didn't feel worth it. It made more sense to explain that I changed my mind, that we would work on ways to make bath time better and not yell at Mommy, and that because it was getting late it was time for everyone to go to sleep.

5. *Validate progress.*

It's always helpful to focus on the positive—not just for your kid, but also for you! It feels nice to add something good to the very stressful mix of tantrum time. So when your toddler takes a step toward completing whatever task you are asking of them, get excited! This might mean intensely validating each tiny move they make closer toward the original goal that started this whole tantrum. Did your toddler's sobs and screams start when you tried to put on their shoes? After some very intense minutes of patient support from you, your little one has calmed down enough for you to bring the offensive, adorable sneakers near them without a complete meltdown. Congratulations, everyone gets a round of applause! Or maybe they're making progress toward a goal that has nothing to do with your original, tantrum-inciting task. Every time my daughter used one of the calming strategies I offered—yes, even throwing a blanket instead of her toy, or screaming into a pillow instead of into my face—I responded with genuine praise.

6. *Invite them to problem solve.*

This is another one where mileage will really vary, especially depending on how worked up your toddler has already become. But it's worth a shot. I ask my daughter for "solutions" all the time, and along the way I feed her possible answers ("Sometimes we set timers and take turns with toys," "I wonder if we could figure out a way to make this Band-Aid look as cool as the unicorn Band-Aids you saw on that commercial"). On many occasions she would join in the problem-solving game. If addressing the problem at hand was too challenging, we pivoted to another task: emotional problem-solving. I would ask my daughter to remind me what we could do "when we get angry," and more often than I expected, she really engaged in, relatively calmly, coming up with a plan.

7. Less is more.

It's okay to talk through things. It's okay to respond attentively, answer questions, give hugs, have conversations, and ditch outdated advice that you must ignore a tantrum. Engaging with your child mid-meltdown does not automatically mean you're reinforcing "bad" behavior. But still, less is often more. I don't ignore tantrums, but I don't negotiate with toddlers—at least not in the way their dysregulation tries to get me to. Avoid getting sucked into tantrum logic-loops. Your little one will argue with all the intensity and manipulation of an expert debater, and you will get nowhere because nothing in the universe can actually motivate them to willingly put away their toys. Short affirmations ("I understand you would rather play. I'll play with you when you clean up. Let me know if you want to work through solutions on how to get that done.") usually make more sense than indulging in counterproductive, irrational conversation.

III. During the peak of a tantrum

It's time to hug it out. Or do the opposite and leave them alone. Or go back and forth. There's no right answer.

This is the hardest part of the tantrum, but also the simplest. Have you ever come home from a terrible day of work, or watched an upsetting movie that triggered something deep inside you, or just reached your emotional limit and, all of a sudden, out of nowhere, you broke down into heaving sobs, experiencing feelings so big you just couldn't keep them inside? I know I can relate, and I know that in those moments of completely overwhelming emotion, there is zero way to reason through it. No thinking, strategizing, or deep breathing can make it go away until it's out. I usually need a big bear hug and someone to just stay with me and make me feel safe. Sometimes I want to be left alone. And I always need to let it out.

Our cathartic cries and emotional outbursts come from the same, primal place as our toddler's meltdown. They're the adult version of a tantrum. We never completely grow out of them, but (hopefully) they occur much less frequently. And the only way to get over them, as an adult or as a child, is to get through them.

So give your kid a hug. Or give them a hundred. Or let them go to their room and yell if they want to. Supporting your child during their dysregulation does not reinforce it, and being a shoulder to cry on is usually a winning strategy. That being said, it's never all-or-none. If you need to briefly tap out and take a break yourself, feel free to do so without any guilt that you're somehow "abandoning" your child. I've had to pause my role as my daughter's emotional regulation guide plenty of times to refocus on my *own* emotional regulation. How could I help her if I lost my own cool? I took plenty of mid-meltdown breaks from my tantrum-coaching to do deep breathing next to my toddler. Sometimes I would even walk away from her (farther from earshot but still within the line of supervision) when I needed a quieter recharge.

And just like disengaging from your child for strategic breaks is more than okay, so is interrupting your child's cathartic moment—especially if there are any concerns for physical safety. Some black-and-white tantrum advice is so focused on allowing this emotional outpouring to proceed without interference that it can seem as if any disruption is harmful. But you can let your child express their emotions without compromising safety. There will almost certainly be times where you need to temporarily disrupt your toddler's catharsis to protect them—and yourself. My daughter knew she could "be angry," but she also knew she wasn't allowed to hurt people. When feelings turned to violence, I held my daughter's hands as I hugged her and calmly but firmly said, "You cannot hit me," while she cried into my arms. Other times I physically picked her up and moved her off the stairs before she raged herself into a fall; I opened her fists and took objects-to-be-thrown out of her hands; and I moved her to cushioned spaces before the headbanging began. I didn't think twice about keeping all our bodies free from harm, and you shouldn't, either. Otherwise, the name of the game was patience. As long as you both are physically safe, you don't have to intervene with anything other than the love they want—and deserve.

THE BOTTOM LINE

5 out of 5 Pediatrician Parents Agree

1. Tantrums are a rite of passage. There are ways to decrease the frequency of tantrums (using the behavioral and emotional strategies in chapter 1), and there are ways to cope when they arise. But there's no way to prevent every single tantrum.

2. Your child didn't read the textbook. Variations in their behavior from the norm, and variations in how they respond to the strategies that you try out don't necessarily indicate something is "wrong" with them—and don't make you a failure.

3. You can and should always seek out expert help with any behavioral question (no matter how small!) as soon as you feel overwhelmed. Your child's expert team will be able to diagnose any issues and provide strategies to help everyone through whatever challenges come your way.

4. Patterns matter more than anything. Any decision is a moment in time, and you can always try a different approach later. There will always be "off" days, and it's okay if you respond differently than you had hoped to—especially if you learn from the experience.

5. Parenting philosophies should fit *your* parenting style, not the other way around.

6. Modern, trending parenting philosophies have a lot to offer but have to be taken with a grain of salt. Ditching strict punishment, focusing on your own reactions, and prioritizing mindfulness all make sense. Extremes like equating praise with parental failure, however, make zero sense.

7. Tantrums have different stages, so you'll need to adjust your coping strategies accordingly. As tantrums are building up—but there's still some intermittent ability to be focused and calm—there's more room to troubleshoot. Some of my favorite strategies are leaning on humor, staying as calm and quiet as possible, giving choices, validating progress, inviting your child to problem solve, and resetting your location or activity.

8. During the peak of a tantrum, your toddler is at their highest level of emotional dysregulation. Try your best not to swim against the tide and instead focus on what you can do: provide a safe space for your toddler to feel their enormous feelings. As long as they are physically safe, do whatever makes sense and help them through it: give big hugs, validate tears, let them scream, give a pillow to throw, give yourself a break, etc.

CHAPTER 3

TOILET TRAINING
The Complex Science of How Toddlers Learn to Pee-Pee and Poo-Poo in the Potty

" I can't wait to toilet train my toddler," said no one ever. As you face new challenges almost daily in preparing your toddler to be a more functioning human in society, helping your kid pee and poop in the potty can be a true pain in the butt. Our vision of toilet training—accidents, limiting outside adventures to avoid the search and use of public toilets, and, of course, toddler tears—can make the hassle and cost of diapering seem like a relative breeze. But while there are almost always stresses associated with this process, the reality is that a lot of the angst is unnecessary. Really. The biggest pains around toilet training are a product of a society that continues to make the basics of parenting overcomplicated. Here's how to take on toilet training with minimal worry and (at least emotional) mess.

If you're reading this book, you're a thoughtful parent filled with thoughtful questions. But when the Wild, Wild West of online advice overwhelms basic instinct, the most important questions sometimes get pushed aside. As always, the crucial question when looking at any parenting topic is *why*. In the case of toilet training, asking "Why toilet train?" starts with a fundamental and almost universally ignored question: Do kids *need* to be toilet trained? The short answer, in the majority of cases, is no.

Most kids will learn how to toilet on their own. Really. There's no science to support the idea that a formal training plan is needed at all. Instead, science shows that norms and strategies around when and how kids learn to toilet independently vary dramatically across cultures, with plenty of children acquiring these skills in an extremely unstructured, deadline-free way.

So why do we toilet train, if it's something that most children will learn on their own? Because society is failing us. A laissez-faire approach to toileting is often impossible in a world where parental support is slim to none. There are lots of reasons that waiting to ditch diapers until your child figures it all out by themself is unlikely to be a realistic option. It could be something as simple as needing to start childcare, with many daycare centers requiring kids to be toilet trained by a certain age. Or maybe your child needs a little extra guidance to stay on track with peers, making the logistics of playdates, travel, and daily life more feasible. Or maybe it's just your preference, and you're sick of diapers, ready to get your toddler's skin rash-free, ditch the search for and use of public changing stations, and keep your wallet a little fatter. Whatever the reason, many parents decide to give toilet training a try, which is more than okay. It may be something you do strictly, not so strictly, try for a hot minute, or ditch altogether. This chapter will give you all the information you need to make that decision—a decision that only *you* can make for your family.

Whenever we talk about individual needs—especially when it comes to behavioral strategies, it's important to take a quick developmental detour. So here's a brief aside. We talk a lot about typical development, and other chapters ("Live and Learn" in this book, "Milestone Madness" from my first book) take a deep dive into the laws of averages, settling on the too often overlooked truth that all kids grow and develop differently. But the topic of atypical development is a big one, and something that's part of my regular clinical work. I treat patients with a host of medical and behavioral conditions, frequently interconnected, which make parenting guidance trickier to sort through. When I say that most children learn to use the toilet without formal training, this generally refers to children without the significant behavioral or medical challenges that many parents have to navigate (on top of the already overwhelming challenges of just being a parent!). It's yet another reason that one-size-fits-all approaches are destined to fail, and why your expertise in your own child will trump any and all advice.

Knowing *why* you're pushing toilet learning along will help you decide which strategies are best to try. Your timeline and motivation are everything. In medicine, we love to say that the answer will "declare itself." Preparation is important, but only you and your child will know, when the time comes, if and when toilet training is something you should pursue. There's no right answer with toilet training—a frustrating but liberating truth that you'll keep front and center as you determine your approach. Don't worry, I'm not here to throw you to the proverbial wolves. There is some research behind toilet training techniques. Let's go through the science, arming you with the knowledge you need to navigate the guidebooks (or not!) and choose the strategy that's right for you.

The Sophisticated Science of Getting Your Kid to "Pee-Pee in the Potty"

Many guidelines on toilet training do have supporting research, but not necessarily the type you'd think. There's a lot of theory, many assumptions, and some real limitations in how we can interpret the body of evidence. Let's break it down in broad strokes.

A 2006 evidence-based report for the Agency for Healthcare Research and Quality (AHRQ) by Terry P. Klassen et al. categorizes toilet training strategies into four founding methods. There are countless toilet training guides, but it's helpful to dive a little deeper into each of these four approaches not only because they are the best studied, but because chances are any approach you come across is a modern version, for the most part, of one of these philosophies.

Child-centered approaches

The first two types of toilet training are considered to be child-centered, which in this case means they are based on a child's readiness. These eponymous approaches from Dr. T. Berry Brazelton and Dr. Benjamin Spock (yup, the very same Spock) are more alike than they are different. Both famous pediatricians built their careers working to dismantle the prevailing strict, behaviorist, prescriptive approaches to parenting that prevailed during their lifetimes. Their overarching philosophies were also extremely similar: nothing trumps common sense, and personal parenting decisions should be individualized, based on parental instinct above expert decree. It should come as no surprise, then, that their toilet training approaches both start by stressing the importance of a child's readiness to engage—something that is determined by physical and emotional milestones and that varies for each child. Once a child shows signs of readiness, Spock and Brazelton propose using gradual methods that are designed for typically developing children, and share a goal of creating individualized, positive experiences. Brazelton asserts that poor experiences with toilet training can lead to lasting issues—fear of toileting, constipation, incontinence, for example. It's a premise that jibes closely to Spock's philosophy that emotionally attuned parenting is the key to raising healthy children.

The details in their timelines and strategies vary slightly. Brazelton focuses on milestones that emerge earlier in most kids (voluntary control over bladder/bowel, following basic directions, rudimentary impulse control, understanding verbal instructions, and a desire to please caregivers), so he suggests starting training around eighteen months. Spock doubles down on the principles of training only when kids are ready, without force, which pushes the start date back to twenty-four to thirty months in his book. He emphasizes that relaxed, pleasant training is the goal, encouraging parents to avoid power struggles and negative emotions as much as possible. Trust your child and be patient—they will let you know when they're ready to learn. According to Spock, reinforcement techniques are okay, but criticism and anger are a no-go when it comes to reluctance, refusal, and accidents. Spock also advises parents to present toileting in straightforward terms, steering clear of anything that frames bathroom behaviors as shameful, dirty, secretive, or mysterious.

Parent-centered approaches

The next two approaches are considered parent-centered because the caretaker steers the ship more than the learner, but other than that, they are, strangely, far more different than they are alike.

The Azrin and Foxx method of "toilet training in less than a day" uses operant conditioning—a principle of behavior psychology that shapes a person's behavior with reward and punishment—to teach toileting behaviors as quickly as possible. It's important to note that the original 1971 study by Nathan H. Azrin and Richard M. Foxx, on which the approach is based, was an extremely problematic experiment conducted on nine severely intellectually disabled adults residing in a facility. The methods were as troubling as the premise. Patients underwent an extreme "training" protocol of reinforcement and punishment with the (successful) goal of transitioning from diapers to independent toileting in a matter of hours. Each participant was placed in a "wet pants" alarm to detect accidents. If none occurred, the participant continued along a strict schedule of being made to sit on the toilet every thirty minutes, pushed to drink fluids every thirty minutes, and getting a food or social activity reward every five minutes. When an accident happened, patients were made to undress themselves, be showered, clean their own urine or stool, wash their own clothing, and be forced to stand without a chair in a one-hour "time-out" without any reinforcement or fluid to drink.

Azrin and Foxx's next study, published in 1973, showed that this type of approach could be used in typically developing toddlers with similar success. This slightly larger study of thirty-four mostly male toddlers took place in the child's home (without any parent or caretaker present!) and used methods strongly echoing those of Azrin and Foxx's previous trial. Participants were shown the steps of toilet training through modeling—for example, a child watched a doll "use" the potty to urinate and then would be guided in wiping, emptying the toilet, flushing, putting the doll's pants back on, etc. To encourage frequent urination, children were pushed to drink fluids every five minutes. Beyond that, the name of the game was reward and punishment. Verbal praise and a child's favorite treat (like chips or candy) were given immediately every time a child took any step toward toileting (pulling down pants, sitting on the potty, peeing in the toilet, etc.). There was also plenty of punishment. For example, accidents earned verbal reprimands, five-minute time-outs (sitting in wet pants with no social interaction), and rapid "practice sessions" running around the house to sit on the toilet until the child showed another "good" toileting behavior that could be reinforced.

Today's Azrin and Fox–esque techniques have modernized a bit. Many of them ditch punishment and instead double down on reinforcement. Most mention readiness but focus primarily on the physical rather than the emotional. They recommend that training begin around twenty months of age, if a child has met milestones such as bladder control, ability to follow instructions, communication ability, independent walking, and picking up objects. Once these basic criteria are met, however, it's still Behavioral Psychology 101. This is why these strategies remain fast and effective, with decades of studies since the original boasting an average time-to-toilet-training of just a few hours. In the end, there are many modern variations. But you can usually classify any method that uses strict behavioral conditioning, focuses on a rigid timeline, and isn't too concerned with a child's emotional readiness as a subtype of the Azrin and Foxx philosophy.

The second "parent-centered" technique, often called the "early-elimination toilet training method," also relies on operant conditioning. But otherwise it has so little in common with the Azrin and Foxx (or any other) toilet training approach that it could, and should, be considered as its own unique entity. This is because the end goal is just having a child *physically control* urination and bowel movements—which, at the age this method is used, just means delay voiding for a matter of seconds and has nothing to do with independent toileting activity. In fact, any independent behavior would be impossible, because the aim of early-elimination techniques is to have infants control elimination by their first birthday. It's a strategy that has been used commonly across the globe—communities in China, Africa, India, and South and Central America employ this as a part of typical child-rearing—and has been gaining popularity in the United States over the past few decades. Training literally starts on day one, with the parent trying to learn patterns of elimination (body movement, muscle tension, facial gestures, noises, etc.) in their newborn. By the time the child is around two to three weeks of age, parents are pros in identifying these cues, and place their baby in a "voiding" position whenever they see one—in North America, this is often holding the child over a sink, toilet, or potty. If a baby pees or poops, parents give a feed, physical comfort, smile, praise, or somehow try to reinforce the behavior. If not, there's nothing to do, and both parent and baby go back to whatever they had previously been doing. There's no punishment for the first year, so if baby doesn't make it to the designated area, it's no one's "fault," and everyone goes back to business as usual. But after that, babies are expected to move themselves away from living areas every time they void or stool. In many of these strategies, accidents in living areas initially get a warning, and repeated accidents result in (often physical) punishment.

And the winner is . . . None of these

But I do have favorites, or at least some clear losers. Let's start with early elimination. It's the odd duck out of these approaches, so much so that most parents, at least in the United States, wouldn't even consider it toilet training. If your goal of toilet training involves some general independence, this method clearly falls short. Trying to toilet train your child before they say their first word will likely lead you down a rabbit hole of wasted time and stress. Instead, you should know what the benefits of this approach actually are: using fewer diapers. That's really it. This leads to a ton of downstream perks, of course. Ditching diapers saves money, keeps products out of landfills, and reduces energy consumption from washing reusable diapers. There are potential health benefits, too. Less diapering means less skin irritation, and diaper use is a risk factor for urinary tract infections. I'm a hospital pediatrician, so I deal with infant and toddler urine infections all the time. I'm all for taking reasonable measures to prevent them, and would love to spare as many little ones from infected bladders as possible. But it's a risk-versus-benefit assessment, like always. It's hard to see how the benefit of ditching diapers, even considering the health benefits, would *universally* outweigh the hassle. What's more, spending all this time and energy in reaching an arbitrary deadline will undoubtedly sap the mojo that you'll desperately need for dealing with toddler dysregulation. And, of course, I'm no fan of punishment, *especially* not physical punishment. If you are looking to reduce diaper use, I think it's okay to explore a modified early-elimination approach (I repeat, no punishment, please!) and make sure you're checking in frequently on the big-picture pros and cons. I know that personally I would never have the bandwidth for anything like this, and even worries about serious infections wouldn't have been reason enough to give it a try. But that's me, and you are you. Explore the options but keep your family's needs front and center.

As for the other three toilet training styles, "child-centered" approaches are the clear winners. Ironically, I find the "child-centered" approaches to be more "parent-centered" than the Azrin and Foxx and early-elimination methods. They allow you to respond to your individual child and empower you to be the best parent you can be in your specific situation. At best, it's unnecessary to stress yourself out with arbitrary deadlines and harsh punishment. I disagree strongly with the premise that there's inherent value in teaching toileting as quickly as possible, no matter what, without considering your particular situation.

At worst, science—and common sense—tells that there is potential for real harm. Your kid is unlikely to be emotionally scarred by a brief stint into punishment-based parenting in an otherwise loving home, but I do agree with Brazelton's assertion that negative toileting experiences can lead to issues down the line. As one example, I've seen cases of severe constipation or incontinence that were triggered, or at least exacerbated, by inflexible, aggressive toilet training. I'm hard-pressed to think of a time when taking a modified "child-centered" route, being flexible with your timeline if possible, and adding rewards for efficiency if your timeline demands this, wouldn't be a better option than Azrin and Foxx–style techniques.

Okay, that's all great, but what should I actually do?

Embracing nuance and ditching the black-and-white is great, but it can be overwhelming. Here are some guiding principles and tangible tools that will help you navigate the online ocean of toilet training advice to create your own personalized, flexible plan.

1. *Remember that toilet training is optional.*

There isn't evidence to support needing toilet training at all. There isn't even expert consensus on basic definitions for "toileting," "toileting success," or "toileting failure." Any guide boasting its scientific superiority is, at best, using psychological principles and evidence of efficacy to make some bold, broad claims.

Looking back on my own experience, I realize that I didn't really toilet train at all. No one is more shocked to hear this than I am; I always thought I would do some sort of formal training. When the spring 2020 lockdown presented the perfect opportunity to stay home and power through an official potty curriculum, I instead pushed it off. At first, it was the stress of frontline-worker pandemic parenting, and I told myself that I'd regroup when the dust settled. But even as we got more used to a stable uncertainty, with ongoing precautions keeping us at home more than we'd like, I found my motivation remained poor. It was a perfect storm of circumstance, personality, and privilege. I had no daycare deadlines, could afford diapers, and was dealing with a happy, growing child who was starting to explore toileting behaviors on her own schedule.

Years before, exhaustion and postpartum depression had launched me desperately into adventures in sleep training. I was more than ready to embrace a behaviorally based training approach to anything that would help me get more rest. But toilet training was different: dirty diapers were annoying, but there wasn't any urgency. The effort of formal training seemed to be more of a hassle than it was worth. I ended up mostly following my daughter's lead, encouraging her interest in sitting on the toilet and building awareness of when she felt the urge to void (or had already had a bladder or bowel movement). I brought some training strategies in, for sure, and there was plenty of verbal praise, lots of Spock-style matter-of-fact bodily discussion, and even some screen time rewards during toilet sessions. We progressed to regular, scheduled sessions sitting on the toilet—known as "timed toilet sits." It's a pediatrician-approved staple of managing and preventing toddler constipation, and only becomes punishment when you use punishment or restraint to make it happen.

In short, we winged it, followed her cues, and were fortunate to find a way to pull it all together (over the course of many months) in time for our reintroduction to society.

2. Keep "readiness" in mind —starting with your child's.

There's no one-size-fits-all answer, and there are a host of interconnected factors that will determine when you start your toilet teaching adventure. While it's ultimately a complicated decision, looking at your child's readiness is a good place to start. Readiness may be something you wait for, but even if you can't wait for your child to declare themselves fully "ready," understanding where your toddler is along that process will help you set expectations and understand some physiological reasons challenges are likely to arise. The 2016 AAP guidelines on toilet training lay out some helpful signs of readiness, starting with these basic physical milestones:

- awareness of the urge to void;
- ability to hold in urine (and, later, stool—although sometimes this happens at the same time or even earlier);
- relaxation of the appropriate muscle groups when sitting on toilet;
- awareness of when bowel and bladder are empty;
- knowing how to take off and put on pants;
- and appropriate hygiene (developmentally appropriate, of course, as you may be helping your child when they shout "Wipe my butt, Mom!" for quite some time).

Additionally, your child will find toilet training easiest once they reach some cognitive milestones—like basic language and communication ability to let you know they need to use the toilet. Furthermore, goal-oriented behavior, memory, and attention (hey there, self-regulation!) will help keep them on track with the task of going to the bathroom. Social and emotional development plays a big role in readiness as well. From ages one to three years, there's a huge shift in toddler psychology. They quickly seek increasing autonomy, take pride in their "mastery" of skills, enjoy social praise, all of which can make toilet teaching something that toddlers actually are motivated to do on their own. It's the scientific reason that, even without formal training, most kids could (and would want to) learn to use the bathroom on their own—on their own timeline and in their own way, of course. We're social creatures, wired to learn the rules of our society and model our behaviors after our caregivers. The desire to ditch diapers, at some point, in some way, is no exception.

3. Zoom out and get a bigger picture of "readiness"—including your own, your family's, and what society imposes on us.

In general, most children achieve their readiness milestones somewhere between two and three years. This is usually when childcare centers either start toilet training children themselves (or see kids eagerly dive in as their already-trained peers show off their skills) or require that parents have their kids fully toilet trained before enrolling. Sometimes, though, deadlines are set too early, defying statistical physiologic norms. And frequently, deadlines are set earlier than *your* child is fully ready. Even the most realistic age-based toileting expectations will be too soon for some kids' physical readiness, and too soon for many more kids' emotional development.

It's something to consider when looking into childcare—if, and this is a big if, that's an option for you. There are plenty of parents who don't have a choice, and the only option is a facility that requires toilet training before their child is fully ready. That's our society, and it's nothing you should feel guilty about. If you end up working on toilet training earlier than you or your child would like, and leaning a bit more heavily into behavioral strategies to achieve this, that's more than okay.

On the flip side, you may, like me, find yourself ditching formal toilet training even if your child is technically fully "ready." That's because *your* readiness matters, too! The age cutoffs certainly aren't based in science, and even the developmental deadlines are flexible. You may end up waiting to embrace toilet teaching until a calmer time in your life, even if your child seems eager to learn. The only real "risks" of waiting too long to start potty pedagogy are potential logistical and social issues—the downside of diapers at home and when traveling, a kid feeling left out or behind their peers if toileting is significantly delayed. But that's highly unlikely to be a meaningful concern if you're staying attuned to your family's needs.

Your strategy has the best chance of working when *you* feel empowered as a parent, and when you have the bandwidth to try it. There is no data that supports crowning any single toilet training method as better than the other. There is a lot of common sense and science, however, that supports putting your own family's needs front and center.

4. The right toilet training method (if you choose any) is the one that's right for you.

There are a range of techniques and timelines that you can choose from when it comes to teaching toileting behaviors.

Modern research and expert consensus remind us that accepted norms for toilet training are based on cultural differences and societal expectations.

If you take the formal toilet training route, starting with a Spock-inspired approach makes a lot of sense. You'll add or subtract as needed, or just borrow a few techniques here and there. The menu of options that "child-centered" philosophies lay out is a much healthier one. You don't have to order everything on the menu, but they're all pretty good choices.

A quick reminder: there are certainly "behaviorist" techniques that can be helpful in your toilet training journey. In this book's first two chapters, we talked about why blanket bans on all behavioral strategies are nonsense. Parenting philosophies that strictly prohibit rewards or even basic praise simply don't have science or common sense behind them. Sticker charts are a staple of my clinical work (getting kids to take medicines is *hard*!) and something I've used plenty of times at home. Reinforcement works; isn't "manipulation" when used thoughtfully as part of a loving, bidirectional parent-child relationship; and may very well make its way into your toilet training routine. Same for the use of dolls and modeling when teaching toileting (or any behavior!). Don't worry about using some of the positive strategies that are associated with these least-favorite approaches. It's okay to ditch the strict timelines, shaky science, and nonsensical punishment and keep a few helpful behaviorist tools in your arsenal.

5. Beware of some red flags.

With countless toilet training guides available, it's impossible to grade each one. Instead, here are some important caveats that will help you decide if a plan is worth trying, if only parts of it make sense, or if it's better to try something else altogether.

One red flag that indicates you might be facing an uphill battle is ignoring the simple physiology we already went over. Deciding to start training before you've seen all signs of readiness is an understandable choice, as long as it's deliberate. But a training guide should acknowledge how readiness plays into the equation, including the emotional readiness that Azrin and Foxx acolytes often ignore. Similarly, anything that's black-and-white ignores your child's individuality. A method that boasts toilet training in a certain number of days will either fail some children by definition, or push some families to the brink with overdetermined, behaviorist extremism in order to achieve these results.

As we also discussed, please steer clear of punishment. Reinforcements are more than fine, and using praise, sticker charts, or even screentime rewards won't take away from all the gentle, mindful parenting you do every day. I'm not a fan of food reinforcement, which is a staple of many behavioral strategies. I'll take tablet time over M&M'S as a reward any day. I have a hard enough time balancing teaching moderation, getting good nutrition, and modeling a healthy relationship with food as it is (we'll dive into that in the upcoming

"Picky Eating" chapter). Using treats as reinforcement turns less nutritious snacks into an emotional prize, rather than part of a varied, un-deprived diet. The feelings and associations edible treats create are intense and easily ingrained. They're hard to backpedal when it comes time to create a lower-stress, holistic approach to how your family interacts with both nutrient- and less nutrient-rich food. It's not the end of the world, but bathroom bonbons are an unnecessary way to further complicate the already challenging task of fostering emotionally and physically healthy eating.

I also stay away from anything that interferes with bodily functions. Messing with your child's physiology is much worse than ignoring it. Some guides suggest it's a good idea to overhydrate your child, increasing urination frequency and speeding up the training process. In the best-case scenario, this is just mean, overfilling your child's bladder when they are learning how to control it and causing stress and discomfort. More dangerously, there could be serious health implications; water toxicity is a rare but life-threatening complication of overhydration, and repeated bladder overdistension can lead to long-term incontinence.

6. Stay flexible.

Accidents happen. Yes, this includes the accidents that lead to soiled pants, floors, car seats, and beyond. It also includes the accidents—misfires, hiccups, learning opportunities, whatever you want to call them—that occur on your toilet training journey. The approach you thought would work best for your family might turn out to be an absolute dumpster fire. Maybe you run into behavioral, medical, or developmental challenges that make strict toilet training impossible, or lead you to push it to a later date. Or maybe the heavens will smile down upon you and your child will display an initiative to ditch diapers before the glitter glue dries on your sticker charts. Either way, stay flexible. You can stop, change, restart, and modify your approach as much as needed. And if you're struggling, get help. Your pediatrician will be there to help you work through the difficulties that arise, diagnosing and treating problems related to urination and bowel function.

Staying flexible also means understanding just how dynamic the roller coaster of toddler toileting can be. Set realistic expectations, and allow for the very common, very healthy variations in how children embrace (or fight against) learning to use the toilet. More often than not the path is winding, with many steps back in between the steps kids take forward. This means that children who display full or near-full control of toileting have regressions and accidents—sometimes with stressors, sometimes with small changes in routine, sometimes for no apparent reason at all. Learning to control urine frequently (but not always) comes first, and making it to the toilet for bowel movements can lag many months! Sometimes it's an inability, as fecal continence develops later than urinary continence for most children. Sometimes it's stubbornness. Children frequently assert control through toileting refusal and can take this to such an extreme that it earns the name "toilet refusal syndrome." In these cases, toddlers simply refuse to poop on the toilet and will instead demand to put on a diaper for each bowel movement. As stressful as this extreme is, it's also a phase—most cases resolve themselves with time, proving just how much of a virtue patience can be (with appropriate pediatrician check-ins, of course).

The list of likely normal variations goes on. Many children stay dry during the day long before they can reliably do so while asleep. Sometimes this is an issue of convenience. If you find that your toilet trained toddler has wet Pull-Ups in the morning, there's a good chance they were able to stay dry overnight but decided to pee in their diaper when they awoke in a lazy, early-morning haze. Other times, nighttime continence physically lags behind. Overnight accidents are the norm, not the exception, after daytime toilet training is complete. This can last for weeks, months, or even years— many kids stay in Pull-Ups up until their fifth birthday and beyond! No matter the situation, remember you're not alone. Your pediatrician will help you decide if any medical issues—constipation is, counterintuitively, a common barrier to staying clean and dry—are at work, or if a prescription for patience is all that's needed.

THE BOTTOM LINE

5 out of 5 Pediatrician Parents Agree

1. Traditional toilet training is optional. Most children will learn how to use the toilet through modeling and gentle guidance without a formal game plan. But there are lots of logistical and personal reasons that can make more structured toilet training an appealing option for your family.

2. There is science behind toilet training techniques. The studied strategies are classified as "parent-centered" or "child-centered." "Parent-centered" techniques and their modern descendants are strictly behavioral. There may be some cases where they make sense to try (like if you have a super-strict toileting deadline), but in most cases I'm not a fan. If you explore them, you'll likely want to modify them. Stay away from imposing punishment, using food rewards, manipulating bodily functions, or pushing beyond developmental readiness.

3. "Child-centered" techniques focus on a child's readiness, use gradual methods, and prioritize making the process a positive experience for everyone. This leads to a lot less stress and thereby—ironically—makes them more "parent-centered" in my book. Using some or all of these techniques can be helpful in teaching toileting behaviors.

4. The "child-centered" strategies I like and personally use are: encouraging interest in toileting behaviors; bringing awareness to bladder and bowel function; using neutral, shame-free language; modeling behavior; pretend play; scheduling "toilet sits"; and embracing nonfood reinforcement when you want to speed up the process.

5. Don't forget to check in on your own readiness. Stay flexible and remember you can always take a break and regroup later. Nothing is all-or-none, and the right method is whichever works best for both you and your child.

6. Toilet training is never a "one and done," even when stricter methods are used. Staying dry at night is something that very frequently takes time—as in, it can be years until you decide your child is ready to sleep without a Pull-Up. Many healthy kids learn to pee in the toilet before they poop there, and sometimes this is so extreme it gets the fancy name of "toilet refusal syndrome."

7. Issues with toilet training are common and usually resolve on their own but can sometimes signal medical issues. The most common one is constipation. When in doubt, make an appointment with your pediatrician to see if any workup (or just expert troubleshooting) is needed.

CHAPTER 4

SOBBING IN THE STAIRWELL

Handling Your Little One's Separation Anxiety—and Why It's Okay for Parents to Cry, Too

Whether your baby was relatively easy to entertain or more high maintenance, there's a good chance they were able to be cared for by others during the first months of their life. Many babies have no discernible preference for a primary caretaker for a whole year (even though they did love you more than anyone else deep down, I promise). Then, somewhere between the very broad range of seven and eighteen months, most babies declare their love for you in very dramatic ways. Separation anxiety is a normal developmental milestone and an important part of their psychological trajectory. No matter how normal it is, though, it can be extremely stressful. I'll help you know what to expect and how to deal so that the anxiety—including your own—stays as minimal as possible.

After a grueling pregnancy, delivery, and postpartum experience, I often "joked" that my daughter's easygoing nature was my reward. She was more adaptable than I was, entertaining herself for hours just sitting in her Bumbo chair and babbling adorably to herself while I took care of around-the-house chores. And when it was time to start daycare around her first birthday, even her teachers were amazed. She let me drop her off without fanfare, smiled the whole day through, and cried exactly zero times. Her teachers said they had never seen anything quite like it.

So when it was time to transition to an older classroom, the screams, cries, and sobs hit me like a punch in the face. I knew that it was normal, even healthy, to have separation anxiety burst onto the scene. Changing classrooms was a big change, but sometimes it doesn't even take a major transition. I knew in theory that, suddenly, my daughter might start to protest being left with caretakers she was already comfortable with. I knew everything was okay; felt my daughter was safe at her very excellent, reputable, monitored daycare; and wanted to handle the meltdowns as another toddler "no big deal." After all, I had to get to work! No time for drama.

That's not what happened, of course, and it turns out that the emotions that were the most challenging to handle were my own. On occasion, after drop-off, she screamed for me, and I hid in the stairwell outside her classroom sobbing. It was the most stressful time since the immediate postpartum, and all my own anxieties came straight up to the surface. My mom guilt, my own memories of childhood anxiety, my instinctive parental worries all rushed into my head and made it impossible to know what to do.

Of course, everything is temporary, especially in the toddler years. The intense pangs of separation stress didn't last forever, and I relied on friends, caretakers, and experts to help us all get through it. I did a lot of reflecting, too, on my own responses and learned so much about how my daughter and I could coregulate our emotions (or not!) along the way.

Let me share those lessons learned, as well as a scientific background on separation anxiety that will help you best prepare for this terrible toddler rite of passage.

The Science of Separation Anxiety

If I hadn't taken college-level child psychology, then continued to study child health and medicine as a career, I think the idea that babies can be so socially chill for months and then suddenly develop a major case of "stranger danger" would seem really weird to me. I mean, when you think about it, it *is* weird. But it mostly makes sense if you take a quick look at typical infant development. A lot of our species' quirky development is a product of our *underdevelopment* in utero. Compared to other animals, humans are born undercooked, with skills and needs more like those they had inside the womb than outside. While some mammals can straight up walk around right after birth, humans remain nearly completely dependent on caretakers for mobility, feeding, soothing, and any chance at survival for months and months. It's fascinating, based on complex evolutionary and biological trade-offs, and simply bizarre.

What does this have to do with separation anxiety, you may ask? Undercooked human babies come with under-cooked baby abilities. Newborns couldn't even have true separation anxiety if they tried. For the first two months, babies often have trouble telling caregivers apart. Yes, they can recognize a mother's smell and sound, bond intensely with primary caretakers like mom, and certainly prefer how some people feel, smell, cuddle, and rock them. But they don't have the skills—both sensory and social—to reliably discriminate between caretakers.

It isn't until two to three months, on average, that a baby's basic social skills emerge. That long-awaited social smile debuts, eye contact and responsive cooing take hold, and we see a shift over the months after this where infants start to con-sistently differentiate between the caretakers around them. This skill takes time to develop. While it does, babies also start to understand their own separateness—the fact that they are their own physically distinct person—and that those other, very beloved, now distinct caretakers can leave them.

To summarize: it takes months for babies to consistently recognize who's who and come to the full realization that the who's who among them can up and leave them. Here's the problem: when these realities kick in—usually around six to nine months—most babies haven't developed "object permanence," the concept that something still exists even when it's not seen or heard. Picture it: you're a baby who has been held, fed, soothed, kissed, cared for nearly around the clock. First you learn how to tell people apart, and as a result create a deep attachment to your A-list circle of caretakers. Then you realize that they can physically leave you, becoming deeply aware of their absence when it occurs. And then, it can take *months* until your brain can accept that even when you can't see, hear, or feel the person you love the most, they haven't completely vanished off the face of the earth.

I don't know about you, but I would certainly cry in that situation. This basic science of how and why babies learn and express "stranger danger" explains why it's a standard, predestined rite of passage. But understanding the neuroscientific origins of this phase is just the beginning. Separation anxiety may come on suddenly, but it rarely goes away as quickly. Part of this has to do with gaining object permanence, a skill that is strengthened gradually rather than an ability that gets turned on like a light switch. And it gets even more complicated: as an understanding of object permanence grows—and even after it's mastered—there is still a world of emotions around separation that need to be navigated. Take a personal example: you may know that your friend is coming back from vacation, but you can still miss them deeply. Replace "friend" with "person I rely on to physically and emotionally survive," throw in some cognitively appropriate doubt that they really are going to come back when they say, and mix it up with a day of never-ending transitions and a near complete lack of control, and you have a sense of what toddlers go through.

Remember, as we reviewed in glorious detail in the first two chapters of this book, the toddler years are a time of non-stop social navigation, exponential developmental growth, and trial-by-fire acquisition of emotional regulation. Even when your toddler understands that you're coming back, managing the transition away from you is *tough*. Oversized reactions are standard for little ones, a parenting principle that can help explain those heartbreaking but completely developmentally normal goodbye sobs.

The separation anxiety off-ramp is a slow and steady one. Navigating the transition from your child's peak separation anxiety to more manageable social stress is a complex, dynamic, and individual journey. In fact, this is one of the major tasks of toddlerhood! Your kid will spend the next years learning to balance the conflicting needs of exploring the world around them with the goal of seeking shelter with trusted caretakers. It's no small feat. As they are better able to manage these opposing goals, they're tasked with even more social and emotional challenges. It's something that you'll be there to guide them through, and it's a choose-your-own-adventure path toward getting there.

There are, of course, resources to help you, and principles to inform your strategies. But there's also a lot of noise, and a lot of groundless guilt. Separation anxiety is extremely stressful—for parents more than anyone! And where there's parenting stress, we know that fear-based, exploitative advice is sure to follow. It's why you'll still find countless sources claiming that even thoughtfully, lovingly proceeding with periods of separation (despite your toddler's protests) is somehow harmful. These claims even cite research in attachment theory, the science behind how animals (including humans) develop secure, lasting bonds with their children. But while guilt-inducing guides might make attachment seem black-and-white, the reality is anything but.

A very brief review of the history of attachment theory helps us understand how we got to the simplistic and problematic advice we still see today. Decades upon decades ago, psychologists preached outrageous, antiquated theories—e.g., mothers are only good for the milk they provide and no better than a food-dispensing machine. It took decades more to correct, then overcorrect, this fallacy. The end result was an also-problematic extreme, birthing an entire movement of "attachment parenting." This philosophy based itself largely on observations—obtained through incomplete study and with dubious methodology—of international communities where practices like baby wearing were the norm. Findings (lots of communities hold, wear, and nurse babies way more than we do in the United States) led to assertions (near-constant baby touching is natural and therefore good), which led to a movement: attachment parenting. This philosophy asserts that parents, usually mothers, must maximize the time they physically hold (and ideally breastfeed) their babies in order to prevent catastrophic psychological outcomes.

Attachment parenting doctrine persists. You'll find all-or-none parenting philosophies that stick to this script more tightly—like prescriptions for nonstop baby wearing, mandatory bed sharing, and breastfeeding at all costs. Some of those same guides ridiculously position separation, especially in the face of anxiety, as literal baby poison. Other times, the attachment undertones are less obvious. If you dig deep enough, you'll find it hiding even in more measured advice. These guidelines assert that, yes, stranger danger is inevitable and separation is allowed, but that pain you feel when your baby cries out for you? It's actually guilt from knowing that every second you spend away from them can permanently damage the bond you share. The attachment-ite subtext is insidious, incorrect, and an effective way to sell products, courses, and subscriptions.

Of course, as always, there's a middle ground. If you're reading this book, you've already committed yourself to creating a loving, secure relationship with your child. You don't need to take a PhD-level dive into attachment neuroscience to feel confident in your ability to provide affection and respond to your child's unique ways of dealing with emotional challenges. The psychology is just here to remind you that attachment is complicated, frequently challenging, and always messy. Separation stress is part of a biologically normal and necessary process of child development, no matter how you slice it.

You, now: *Phew, thanks, got it! I feel better!*

You, a few moments later: *Wait . . . there are super convincing posts and videos still assuring me that separation from my kid is bad and there will be long-term damage! Are you sure it's okay to be my own human person?*

Sheesh, it's rough out there! The internet really is trying to make parenting impossible. It tells you the safe, scientific, sensible choices that you (the expert in your child!) make are somehow wrong.

They aren't. I can confidently say that anyone who claims to have a one-size-fits-all answer to secure parent-child attachment is missing the mark. We know some of the *basic* ingredients that are nonnegotiable. You need to feed your child, keep them clean, provide shelter, and have a caring person care for them every day. The strong science we have behind this comes from tragedy—early animal studies showing that monkeys removed from their moms and fed with wire contraptions became horribly depressed, horrific cases of abandonment in orphanages, and case studies of abuse, to name a few. Prescriptions for nonstop baby wearing, moms who never work or leave the house, mandatory bed sharing for years and years are all based on theories. And they're limited theories based on limited studies. Most attachment-informing anthropological studies were observations of global communities using very unrigorous methodology, and done by researchers who didn't really care about fully understanding their subjects.

What this means for *you* is that the "scientific" benefits of affection and love are *real*. Being a generally responsive, attentive parent is—no surprise—good for your child! But the "scientific" benefits of an attachment doctrine don't exist. There is no evidence that thoughtful, temporary, planned separation between parent and child is harmful. Instead, we have science that shows the opposite. It's no surprise that most of this attachment parenting messaging has been directed at mothers, usually as part of a thinly veiled, misogynist attack on women working and spending time outside of the home. So scientists decided to test this anti-feminist theory, and quickly debunked it. There's a rich body of evidence now demonstrating how early childcare has *no* link to adverse outcomes later in life. Similarly, there's no data (or common sense) to support claims that a certain amount of baby wearing, bed sharing, breastfeeding, or any specific bonding tool is better than any other. These are *tools*, part of a bigger picture of attachment, and only help promote your connection to your child if they help you feel connected to your child.

Periods of separation aren't dangerous. And in most cases, some amount of separation anxiety also isn't dangerous. But it *is* stressful. We do have research showing that kids frequently struggle when transitioning to a new childcare, with some studies even showing elevations in the stress hormone cortisol during this period. Don't get it twisted: this does *not* mean some serious, physical harm is occurring.

The cortisol levels aren't very high, nothing like those we see with severe neglect or abuse. Cortisol is an adaptive hormone, one that is elevated periodically throughout our life to make sure our bodies have what they need to respond to threats. Short, mild elevations of these hormones—when paired with a supportive relationship with a caretaker—are part of what scientists call "positive stress." Many argue it's an important part of children's development and a necessary step in establishing a healthy stress-response system. And, importantly, these cortisol elevations decrease after a brief period of adjustment.

What all the studies show, when taken together, is that separation anxiety is common, stressful, and temporary. You can ditch any worries over long-term damage and focus instead on managing the anxiety—both your toddler's and your own—as best you can. Remember, even if you're not going the full-time childcare route, helping your child learn that they can have some separation from you is a *good* thing. Toddlers are tasked with trying to achieve that seemingly impossible balance between attachment and autonomy, learning how to navigate a world with increasing independence while still running back to you as a home base. It's another reason why any extreme philosophy just doesn't make sense. Like everything, separation is a mixed bag, an emotional, challenging road bump that's also an opportunity for both you and your toddler to acquire skills and strengthen your evolving relationship.

This, Too, Shall Pass. But How?

Hopefully you feel completely confident in your childcare setup, knowing you've sorted through the full spectrum of risk and benefit and that separation anxiety is a developmentally normal stressor, not a sign of failure.

But maybe "stressor" is an understatement. It was for me, and my personal suffering lasted longer than it needed to. So let's break down how you'll create your own loving, guilt-free playbook if and when the stairwell sobs come your way.

1. Lean on your support team.

As challenges emerge—or if you have the bandwidth to preempt them—your childcare providers will be a tremendous resource. Not only do they have amazing tips and tricks from their years of expertise, but there's evidence that partnering with other caregivers to create a customized transition game-plan leads to better outcomes.

There's still a lot of debate around exactly how to stage an optimal adjustment to an outside childcare setting. Some qualitative studies suggest gradual methods might be easier, but evidence is limited. And, in the United States, at least, less-than-acceptable parental leave means that phasing your child into daycare may be impossible for you, and likely something your daycare doesn't even have as an option due to the lack of societal support needed to make it sustainable. But even if a gradual transition is out of the question, there are plenty of evidence-based strategies your childcare provider will be happy to partner on. When parents stay involved in the process—and, most important, work with a key person (like a single teacher) to create a transition plan—the process is easier. Even if you can't start with reduced daycare hours, adopting a "key person" approach and viewing it as a group assignment that you tackle together will help mitigate a lot of stress.

2. Pour your energy into the times you're together.

As I leaned into the quality-over-quantity approach to parenting—finally giving myself some permission to feel pride in the positive bond I made with my daughter and not obsess over the hours we were apart—I tried to make some deliberate, psychic shifts. When I was away, she was safe and still cared for. No need for guilt. But if I wanted to feel I was strengthening our bond, I could work on strengthening our bond. No pressure, just love. Extra snuggles, more time putting down my phone and playing together, extra effort in engaging in the activities that made *both of us* happy. And when I wanted to feel that I was more concretely addressing separation anxiety, I was a little less subtle with my messaging. We read books on the topic, and I frequently replaced the plots of my less-than-favorite picture books with made-up tales of a devoted working mother who always, always came back for her baby.

This is all optional, and something I did as much for me as for her. It was a way for me to stay connected, to focus on the positive, to channel my energy into that secure attachment we had already forged. Which, as you might imagine, makes separation less stressful. In those hormone studies we went over, researchers have found that cortisol elevations are *much* higher in children with insecure attachment styles than in their securely attached counterparts.

3. Create a routine, make it deliberate, and make it yours.

Creating a goodbye routine might be simple—a quick hug, kiss, or wave is all some toddlers need. But if transitions come with more fanfare, it can be helpful to have a more personalized song and dance. This might be a literal one, like in my case. As we ramped up in our separation struggles, a tune from a long-forgotten VHS tape of kid songs from the 1980s, which ran on repeat during my childhood, popped into my head. With every transition I sang an updated remix, hugging and rocking her to a silly melody with sillier lyrics promising to return and assuring that I would never, ever forget her.

As we talked about with "key person" strategies, there's still lots of debate as to what makes a "good" transition. A perfectly planned acclimatization is a privilege. We know that not everyone has the time or resources to stage a stepwise phase-in process. If you're one of the many who doesn't have the ability or energy to do this, that's okay. There are lots of ways to work with your childcare provider to make the transition smoother. Your child will *not* be traumatized because you didn't start them with shorter hours, stay in their classroom with them, or do a longer period of joint sessions with you and a nanny.

The reason I'm talking, again, about how gradual approaches can be helpful is to remind you that, like always, there's an equally incorrect assertion in the opposite direction. I can't count how many times I was told (by nonexperts) to just say goodbye and bounce. Don't get me wrong—I'm a fan of making sure your kid knows you're leaving (ghosting is never cute), and I also love a well-planned, short transition. Just stay away from the extremes. You don't have to phase your child into their surroundings minute by minute, hour by hour, day by day. You also don't have to yell "Bye!" and run out of the room. You'll find a middle ground between sprinting away from a screaming toddler and sinking into an amorphous, indefinite, anxiety-affirming group meltdown. Talk to your "key person," and you'll find a routine that splits the difference and serves everyone best.

4. If it's not manageable, ask an expert!

And if you don't find your groove—or if the process is lasting a bit too long or becoming overwhelming—seek help! Finding a true expert (like a child psychologist or family therapist) who can work to give you direct, individualized guidance is a sign of strength. Your pediatrician is there, too, and can help connect you with resources like these. You shouldn't—and don't—have to go through it alone.

If it doesn't feel normal, healthy, or even manageable, seek help!

5. Take care of yourself.

It's trite, but it's true. And it's all too easy to forget. Your health matters—not just because you're worth taking care of, but because it directly promotes your child's health! When it comes to modeling emotional regulation, we know that parents play a critical role. Self-regulation is a process, one that's facilitated by how children see it around them. Your own emotional responses need to be attended to. Honoring your feelings and working on your own resilience will reap enormous benefits.

Remember, self-efficacy is a scientifically proven parenting asset. If you feel confident in your choices, this will make things easier for everyone and carry long-term psychological benefits. Easier said than done, I know. I found the hardest part of our separation journey wasn't the physical separation, it was the task of emotionally separating myself from my daughter. I was so focused on my daughter's reactions (understandable) that I didn't realize how much my *own* contributed to our struggles. I worked hard to take a step back and figure out how much of her anxiety was hers, and how much was my own projection of what I "felt" she was experiencing. It's still super hard to untangle whose feelings are whose, what worry comes from what, and who really needs to learn to tolerate a little more distress. Be patient, reflect, regroup. Separation anxiety is the beginning of a new phase of autonomy—for both you and your child. You'll both learn how to be separate people, while still knowing you'll always be there, unconditionally, for support. It's a tough task, but worth the effort, I promise.

"No, Just Mommy!"

A lesser-known fact about separation anxiety is how it might find its way into your home. No, not just when you leave your child with a childcare provider. Even wilder, your child may very well channel their newfound, intense preference for a single caretaker into day-to-day activities, even when you're right there, in front of them, absolutely going nowhere.

It's called caretaker preference, and it caught me totally by surprise. Around the time of peak separation anxiety, I found my daughter wanted to be around me all the time. Sometimes it seemed logical: she rejected my desire to leave the house for brief periods, wanting to continue the near-constant physical attachment that we both adored. Sure, continuous snuggles could be exhausting—plenty of people get "touched out" for much less, and this makes you *no less* of an amazing, loving parent—but it was the next step that finally tested my patience. With caretaker preference, another beloved caretaker could be standing just millimeters away, and a toddler will insist, instead, that the preferred caretaker do everything. And I mean *everything*. Mommy's in the bathroom? That's okay, I'll just barge in and ask her to put a straw in my cup. Mommy's on a phone call? That's no reason to ask Daddy, who is literally holding me, for a diaper change. I coped with attempts at humor, nearly ordering myself a custom T-shirt with "No, just MOMMY!" printed on the front.

Knowing it's a phase can help. It *is* a phase and should get better with time. But sometimes you can't wait. It's okay to be overwhelmed and tap out as much as you need. As the preferred parent I was exhausted, and even resentful. I *knew* that other caretakers wanted to help, but it was hard for them to recognize when they should step in. I'm sure it was frustrating for them, too, and if I had been in that situation I would imagine, as irrational as it seems, that my feelings might even have felt hurt, instinctively sad that my child didn't want *me*!

Besides patience and grace—and a lot of caretaker debriefing—I found a few scripts to be helpful. Frequently I responded to my daughter's constant requests with "Honey, Mommy loves you so much and I love helping you, but sometimes I need help, too. Let's ask Daddy to do this for you. Can you help me by asking him?" Not a silver bullet, but a huge help. Like with all parenting scripts and toddler behavioral challenges, you'll take it one day at a time, acknowledging just how challenging this phase is while remembering that, like everything else, this too shall pass.

THE BOTTOM LINE

5 out of 5 Pediatrician Parents Agree

1. Separation anxiety is normal and healthy, a product of our evolution and development. It can help ease the stress to remember that this is an adaptive phase that usually resolves by itself over time.
2. Remembering it's normal doesn't take away the stress entirely, though, and there are ways to cope. Partner with your support team; caretakers and daycare teachers are ready to share expertise and create a game plan! There's no one right way to carry out a transition, but being deliberate and coordinated is the key to success. Double down on consistency in routine—with separations and other transitions—as much as possible.
3. When the emotions hit hard—your emotions, that is—take stock of your responses. Whether it's solo reflection or a good therapy session, you'll find that taking time to unpack your own thoughts and feelings can help reframe your entire approach.
4. If you have the bandwidth and want to "do something," try to pour leftover energy into the "together" times. Make up special songs, handshakes, and goodbye routines in advance. Practice them through pretend play, read books, or watch shows on the subject, and keep up all the great emotional-regulation work you started after reading this book's first chapter.
5. Attachment theory has science behind it. But extreme philosophies and the guides that borrow from them are grounded in exploiting parental guilt, not actual data. Proceeding with periods of separation in the face of screams and protest—when done thoughtfully and lovingly—will not permanently harm your child.

6. Seriously. Research shows that early childcare has *no* link to adverse outcomes later in life. Studies also show that prioritizing time together, creating secure attachments, and embracing strategies like a "key person" to help in the transition period all make the process easier.
7. Caretaker preference is normal, temporary, and very annoying— both for the preferred and not-preferred caretakers. Caretaker coordination and communication are key. The preferred caretaker can stockpile a few scripts to easily tag out of tasks, and the non-preferred caretaker can focus on how and when to jump in proactively.

CHAPTER 5

CREATURES OF HABIT

Tackling Thumb-Sucking, Pacifiers, and Other Veritable Toddler Addictions

After doing your research (hopefully my first book, *Parent Like a Pediatrician*, helped!) and weighing the risks and benefits, you decided to take the plunge and introduce a pacifier to help your baby self-soothe, and it has been a godsend. You gave your child their binky without guilt, knowing you'll be able to help them quit. Except, now that it's time to quit, the task doesn't seem quite as simple as you thought it would be. Or maybe pacifier addiction isn't your issue, and your toddler's thumb-sucking is what's causing stress. Or maybe it's an entirely different habit—just wait until we go over some of the possibilities—that your little one just can't kick. Never fear, this chapter is here.

No matter what habit consumes your child's daily routine, you'll be able to make it to the other side. Sometimes it makes sense to intervene, and other times the truth is that everyone will be happier (and the issue will resolve itself more easily) if you just let it run its course. Let's break down some of the common toddler behavioral quirks and compulsions you'll encounter, and as always, expert tips in how to deal with them.

Some Favorite Habits and Some Targeted Tips for Managing Them

1. Pacifiers

Like many, I made the decision to embrace binky use for a variety of reasons—potential SIDS (sudden infant death syndrome) protection first and foremost. But in my under-supported, overwhelmed postpartum state, I wasn't going to say no to any tool that could soothe my baby. I've said it once and I'll say it again: pacifiers work, *can* be part of a breastfed baby's routine if used appropriately, don't convincingly cause ear infections or permanent dental issues, and shouldn't be a cause of parental anxiety or guilt.

There *is* a downside to how well pacifiers pacify: it sure can be hard to quit them. It doesn't help that countless sources still push a mandate to stop pacifier use as early as six months, or more commonly around one year (a childless pediatric version of myself was regrettably guilty of this!). Even if you tune out the noise and remember that the use of an unsweetened paci is pediatrician mom–approved *throughout* the entire toddler years, you still might need some help quitting when the time comes. That time might come when your child is ready to enter preschool, or it may come sooner. In my case, I found a good time emerged around my daughter's second birthday, when our life was relatively stable. I was also sick of bringing binkies everywhere and looked forward to a paci-free photo of my adorable child.

How did we do it? I knew there were lots of options, and just like sleep training, toilet training, or any other behavioral intervention, the secret to success was parental comfort and confidence. After two years, my husband and I had figured that, generally speaking, gradual methods were our jam. Successful Ferberizing and an ongoing laissez-faire approach to potty education had built our confidence in all things slow-and-steady. So, I knew instinctively that transitioning pacifier use strictly and solely for bed and naptime was the best first step—with her nanny and daycare teachers helping to keep this consistent rule. There were some initial mini-meltdowns and the occasional tantrum, but in all honesty, they blended into the ongoing ebbs and flows of normal toddler dysregulation. Within days, my daughter knew that binkies were for bedtime and simply stopped asking for her paci at other times.

Just over a month later, after needless worrying over the seemingly inevitable nightmare of removing her nighttime pacifier, we took the final leap. We thoroughly prepared her for days in advance—"Now that you're a big kid we need to give your pacifiers to the other babies to use and you'll be able to sleep on your own and be just as safe as always"— then one night simply put her to bed empty-mouthed. Prepared for endless screams, I was met with whines and whimpers that quickly subsided into slumber. We repeated our pep talk for a few more nights until the memory of her precious piece of plastic seemed to have completely vanished.

It wasn't a fluke. Since then I've counseled countless parents on how to use this strategy to kick their little ones' binky habits, with similar success. There are, of course, other approaches, and if a slower or faster version of this game plan is more aligned with your family's needs (including your own timeline), that's more than okay. Modifications to this method will map out just like any other behavioral intervention: you can go faster to the point of suddenly removing all pacifiers much like "cry it out" sleep training, or you can phase out pacis even more slowly than I did. With older kids, social cues from paci-free peers may make your kid a more willing participant in weaning—like with child-centered toilet training. I say *more* willing, not willing, because toilet training this ain't. Meaning, pacifiers are indeed addictive, and your toddler is less likely to abandon their binky on their own than they are, say, to seek toilet learning just because it's what all the cool kids are doing these days.

When the time is right, take that paci away. Slowly, quickly, gradually, tomorrow or today. Use the words that help guide you and your child through it together. And don't obsess. Overcomplicated methods are at best an unnecessary stress. Some parents replace pacifiers with a blanket, toy, or other transition object, which is fine but definitely not needed, and does replace one dependence with another, albeit much more desirable, one. I'm not a personal fan of branded "pacifier-weaning systems" that give your child a shorter-tipped paci every few days until they realize they're sucking on nothing and give up. These systems aren't dangerous, they're not that expensive, and some parents find them really helpful. So if it's something you want to try, go for it. However, my preference has been to start with a more collaborative, straightforward approach. There just isn't any compelling evidence that these devices work better than a strategic, simple wean, and my instinct is to avoid overcomplicated, mildly deceptive techniques if there's an effective alternative. Cutting holes in pacifier tips (which interferes with suction and makes them less appealing to use), on the other hand, is something to avoid. The sharp edges on cut pacifiers can hurt little mouths, and plastic pieces can even fall off and be choking hazards.

2. Thumb-sucking/finger-biting/blanket-chewing

Congratulations! You successfully weaned your little one from their pacifier and are continuing to just nail this whole parenting thing. Nothing ahead but sunshine, blue skies, and—seriously, my love, are you really going to put your fingers in your mouth all day? In a cruel twist of fate, it turns out that the hard work of kicking a paci addiction can be the easier part of this journey. Many children whose pacifiers are taken away quickly replace this habit with another, swiftly learning to suck thumbs, fingers, or chew on whatever is in sight. Others have been doing this for months, even years, no matter how much parents pushed a pacifier in its place.

Don't worry, there's good news: you'll get to the other side of this, and there are strategies that can help you get there. The bad news is that, unlike with pacifiers, stopping nail biting and finger sucking isn't as easy as just taking an object away. Instead, you'll find a whole wide world of products and guides that claim to be the key to kicking this trickier habit. Which tools make sense, and which ones can you ditch? It's time to dive in, sort fact from fiction, and share my safe, realistic, scientific approach.

Are there any evidence-based strategies to kick these nasty habits? The short answer is, thankfully, yes. As with all of pediatric medicine and especially behavioral pediatrics, there isn't as much data on this topic as we would like. But there are studies that serve as a good jumping-off point, giving a comprehensive overview of the techniques that are out there and whether they even work.

A 2015 Cochrane review (the gold standard for meta-analysis) is a good place to start our discussion. This article scoured the available literature to see what trials exist on "non-nutritive suck cessation"—a fancy phrase to describe how to stop thumb-sucking, finger-biting, blanket-chewing, pacifier use, etc. They found six trials that met their search criteria, and note that our ability to interpret and compare results is very limited due to the methodology (i.e., how the studies were designed). Two trials had low-quality evidence that dental devices were effective. There's a wide variety of orthodontic devices that can be used to kick oral habits, too many to go over one by one here. But it's important to know a few things about them. Often called palatal arches or palatal cribs, these contraptions all work by making it harder or less desirable for a toddler to suck on their fingers. There's a huge world of difference, however, between the various types. Some are removable and can be taken out throughout the day, while others are fixed in place by a dentist and designed to stay in place for months. They also come in various designs, ranging from the kind that serve as gentle reminders when a child's thumb hits mouth metal to the kinds that physically block the mechanics of thumb-sucking or—my least favorite—have something sharp to make the prospect of putting a finger in the mouth unpleasant. As for nondental interventions, this review found two similarly limited trials that showed short-term effectiveness of using positive or negative reinforcement strategies. In conclusion, there is some, limited, low-quality evidence that reinforcement, palatal cribs, or arches are more effective than doing nothing at all.

As far as data goes, this is pretty unimpressive. Other studies help round out the body of evidence: some look at specific devices like those cribs and arches, others look at elbow guards, an immobilizing cuff that physically restricts the movement of your child's thumb into their mouth. In general, the trend is that they help break the habit more than doing nothing. The limitations to these studies are significant, and it's hard to take much from them. Newer studies (some even less generalizable, including case studies), point toward another direction. Simple interventions like placing a reminder sticker on a child's thumb—that's literally it, a doctor just says it's a special sticker not for chewing and the toddler decides if they'll abide—are gaining traction. Positive reinforcement, reminders, and gentler behavioral strategies have also been described in the literature and have plenty of success stories. All in all, the data is limited but confirms that there are various interventions that may be effective in stopping your toddler's thumb-sucking.

That's some nice science you got there, but what should I do?

Even if we had better data (which we hopefully will one day!) to support the effectiveness of one strategy over another, it's important to take a step back. Looking at scientific evidence—especially evidence that just focuses on how well strategies work and not all the other messy big-picture risk versus benefit assessment—is just the first step. The more important task is deciding what you should do to help your specific child (and if you should intervene at all).

We talked about how, with pacifiers, the risks aren't high enough for a total ban. Specifically, orthodontic effects are usually reversible if kids stop using them around age three, or even age five according to some experts and studies. This is the same for thumb-sucking—it isn't until kids pass the toddler years and permanent dentition starts to enter the equation that I bring this worry into the risk/benefit equation. Of course, there are other potential harms with this habit. Social stress from being a prolonged thumb-sucker is unlikely at this young age but something that could be a consideration. More common and significant? Blisters, infections, and a wide world of finger woes that can be painful and tricky to manage. This is the most frequent reason I find the risk-versus-benefit equation tips in favor of an earlier push to help your child stop sucking their thumb. When hand problems come into play, a more structured intervention can make a lot of sense.

Still confused? Not sure how to make the best decision for your family? I got you. Here's the approach I take when counseling parents on kicking finger-chewing habits.

My Stepwise Approach to Thumb-Sucking

*Step 1: **Do nothing.*** If you haven't yet been thrust into the world of finger infections, and there aren't any other serious harms visible, it's usually best to just let your one-, two-, or three-year-old do their finger-sucking thing. There's a good chance that it will stop on its own, and that any push to end it earlier will cause unnecessary stress.

If you're still feeling antsy, or just want to ever-so-gently push things along, it's fine to try an alternative comfort measure. Lots of kids put their fingers in their mouths less frequently when they have a blanket, toy, or toddler-safe fidget object as an alternative. Remember, whatever object you choose may become a deeply prized possession. Be ready to have that lovey with you at all times—and likely deal with some major meltdowns when you accidentally forget it at home.

*Step 2: **Do something.*** If your kid is older, or some of those physical harms of constant finger-chewing are starting to pop up, there are things you can do. Those interventions we talked about can be really effective. Which ones you use, as always, depends on your style and your child's response. But just as important is remembering the big-picture risk versus benefit.

A lot of the "less invasive" methods are often just as effective as the fancier devices, and in the majority of cases it's worth it to give those a try first. Giving gentle reminders throughout the day is technically an intervention—and can be an effective one. Positive reinforcement—starting with verbal praise, but leading to giving rewards if the need arises—is a nice next step. I really dig that sticker-on-the-thumb approach, which is sort of in between these two approaches; it's a visual reminder, and if you wanted to add a reinforcement component you could give praise or even a nominal prize if your kid keeps it on the whole day. Punishment doesn't make sense, so keep the reinforcement positive if that's the route you choose.

*Step 3: **Get help.*** Most thumb-sucking will fade away on its own, or with the gentler strategies in step 2. But if you find yourself with an older kid who just cannot stop eating their fingers, and you know there will be (or already is) social and medical fallout if the habit continues, it's okay to want to do more. As always, your pediatrician is your partner, and making an appointment just to discuss this issue and create a game plan is a winning strategy.

If you're at the point of more invasive intervention, deciding there will be real benefit is more important than ever. Make sure it's something that's bothering them more than it's bothering you before diving into the world of habit-breaking devices.

The least invasive of the bunch is nail polish or other bad-tasting, topical treatments that deter a child from eating their fingers. It's probably where I would start, but plenty of parents don't like the idea of painting something gross on their child's nail (understandable), and plenty of children (like five-year-old me) are so addicted to nail biting that bitter polishes become an acquired taste.

Palatal arches and cribs are often effective, but of course it's a bigger intervention, especially the type that are implanted for months. It's not a definite no for me (I would always start with a removable one, and would never try one designed to cause physical discomfort). But the benefits of stopping thumb-sucking quickly would have to be significant for me to want to put a dental device in my child's mouth. Elbow guards are a clearer no as far as I'm concerned. They make it look as if your toddler has an orthopedic injury—an incredibly visible, public, and medical way to pathologize a normal toddler habit. They also limit mobility (intentionally, to stop your child from accessing their thumb), which just doesn't make any sense for play and development. I'm hard-pressed to think of a situation where I'd choose this intervention.

3. Self-gratifying and exploratory behaviors (a.k.a. welcome to the wondrous world of toddler masturbation)

Yes, you read that right. In this wonderfully sex-positive and anatomically correct world, our society is finally starting to catch up to the fact that body exploration and sexuality are totally normal and totally worthy of talking about without fear or shame. But did I really just say that toddlers masturbate?

Before becoming a hospital pediatrician, I wouldn't have believed this either. In fact, I didn't. In residency, I cared for an adorable two-year-old who was admitted for overnight EEG monitoring (checking a person's brain electricity with stickers to look for seizures). Her parents wisely brought her to the doctor because they noticed the child making "abnormal movements." The only way to make sure these movements weren't seizures was to see what an EEG recorded when the movement happened. Fortunately, we captured an episode quickly. And fortunately, it was *not* a seizure. Her brain waves were totally normal, and the seasoned pediatricians and pediatric neurologists recognized quickly that her movements were normal—and self-stimulatory.

This wasn't a one-time thing. I soon became well-versed in the occasionally awkward but always reassuring "your kid does *not* have any serious brain conditions, but they are, indeed, masturbating" talk. Most parents are as surprised as I was when I first learned this was really a thing. Let's review the common, normal phenomenon of childhood masturbation and how to deal.

So, what is childhood masturbation? The common-sense definition is that it's pretty much what it sounds like. The scientific definition is that childhood masturbation is any genital self-stimulation by children, and this includes infants (age birth to one) and toddlers (ages one to three). In these younger ages, manual stimulation is less common than other behaviors, like pressing onto surfaces and placing legs around crib slats. This is why it's so often confused with other things. Movements of legs around crib slats can indeed look like seizures, and some positions make it easy to confuse with abdominal pain or constipation. It can be tough even for professionals to diagnose without some additional investigation, so don't worry about sorting through it on your own. You can always ask your pediatrician to help you make the official diagnosis.

Is this really normal? Is it common? Yes and yes. There's a world of emerging and compelling evidence showing us just how normal and common this phenomenon is. One of the most famous studies comes from William N. Friedrich et al. in 1998. It found that, consistent with earlier research, there were a broad range of sexual behaviors that appear in children, at various ages, and in various frequencies.

Self-stimulation, a.k.a. childhood masturbation, was one of the most common ones.

How common, you ask? In the study's cohort of two- to five-year-olds, they found that 15 percent of girls and 26 percent of boys stimulated their genitals in public, while 43 percent of girls and 60 percent of boys did so at home. Age five seemed to be the peak of this behavior, especially the public component. It makes sense: as kids learn more about social norms and behavioral expectations, overt self-stimulatory displays become more contained.

Since this defining study, evidence continues to support that body exploration, leading to the discovery of pleasurable areas, then leads to the common, healthy phenomenon of childhood masturbation. Sometimes it's used as a self-soothing behavior, meaning that you'll see it more after a life change or stressor. But plenty of times it's just something that toddlers do. Who would have thought?

So, what should I do about it?

The short answer is: nothing. Expert consensus is to definitely not punish or discipline children who explore self-stimulatory behaviors. For toddlers, trying to get them to stop it is usually an uphill battle at best and counterproductive at worst. If there's no downside to this normal behavior, drawing negative attention to it only opens the door to pathological views on bodies and sexuality. Instead, try to focus on what you can do. In the upcoming chapter "Brave New World," we'll go over why diving into touchy topics like anatomy and sexuality is a hard but important task. You'll model healthy viewpoints, open dialogue, and give your child the tools they need to learn about sex without shame or judgment. If you're worried about anything, or just want help in handling this surprising but normal phenomenon, seek an expert! Developmental psychologists have lots of resources (in person and online), and your pediatrician will work to get you the information you need.

Observing, discussing, and navigating sexual behaviors in children is an understandably touchy topic. As a savvy parent, you may be wondering if there ever is a time where sexualized activity is a red flag, or at least a possible cause for concern. The answer is yes, but it's of course complicated. The definition of what is age-appropriate and normal can vary among communities and families, and depends on cultural norms. It's important not to paint too broad strokes, but there are some guidelines that can help distinguish between behaviors that are more likely to be healthy and others that aren't. Sexual behavior that is more likely to be linked to inappropriate activities or abuse is the type that mimics adult sexual behavior—that is, things beyond self-stimulation by pressing against things or using hands. Another potential red flag is when the behavior is obsessive to the point of interfering with daily life. This doesn't mean that abuse is the definite cause, but it does make sense to talk to your pediatrician about how to rule this out. Frequent genital stimulation can also be related to medical issues like skin inflammation, urine infections, or, as we mentioned, triggered by stressors. It makes sense to worry most about recognizing signs of abuse, but really any concern is reason enough to call your pediatrician. It's what we're here for.

When it comes to toddler habits, nothing is more important than picking your battles. Before you spend too much energy trying to change what's going on, ask yourself if it's really a problem. Maybe there are real harms (repeat skin infections are a total bummer) that make the effort worth it. But maybe things are pretty much fine. Or at least fine for now. Almost all toddler habits evolve with time (masturbation becomes private, *phew*, and thumb-sucking might turn into nail-biting no matter how hard you intervene), and many will simply disappear on their own. If a habit isn't hurting your kid, it's more than okay to decide to deal with it later.

THE BOTTOM LINE

5 out of 5 Pediatrician Parents Agree

1. Before you dive in to troubleshoot your toddler's latest habit, take time to reflect if it's really a problem—and if it's something you need to address right now. Most habits go away with time, and with minimal (or no) intervention.

2. Pacifier addictions are hard to kick, and it's common to want to encourage your toddler to stop sucking on their binky before they're completely ready. You can plan a paci wean that's as fast or slow as makes sense for you. Pacifier weaning systems are probably safe but frequently unnecessary. Avoid cutting holes in pacifiers, which carries more risk than benefit.

3. Thumb-sucking, nail-biting, and finger-chewing often resolve on their own, in their own time. Watchful waiting or gentle reminders are usually the best starting strategy. If these habits are persisting, or leading to hand/dental issues, chat with your pediatrician. Usually a sticker chart or other reinforcement strategy is the next step.

4. If sticker charts, rewards, and reminders aren't cutting it, there are other more intense habit-breaking interventions. Make sure to check in with your pediatrician before diving in. Bad-tasting polishes might be an option, and (removable) dental devices are something you'll want to explore with a qualified professional. I'm still hard-pressed to think of a situation where an elbow guard that restricts mobility (and looks like an injury!) makes sense.

5. Toddler masturbation is, remarkably, extremely normal. If you have any concern at all, check in with your pediatrician. Underlying issues like urine infection, stressors, sleep issues, and abuse, are possible but unlikely to be the cause of typical toddler self-stimulatory behaviors.

6. Avoiding punishment and interventions that manipulate body movements or activities is generally a good idea, especially when it comes to dealing with toddler habits.

PART TWO

EATING +
SLEEPING

CHAPTER 6

MILK MONEY

The Truth About Toddler Formula, Extended Breastfeeding, and the Nutrition Growing Bodies Actually Need

You made it! Your baby has passed or is near their first birthday. The infant days are over, and toddler time is officially here. For all the behavioral stresses that this older age brings, there are undeniable joys. New feeding habits *should* be among these excitements. It's complicated, for sure. Change is always hard, and if you're on an evolving breastfeeding journey this can be emotional in all directions. The shift from bottle to sippy cup and solid food is a milestone to be processed as well. It's messy, and not just because of the spaghetti your toddler will inevitably throw across the room.

It's not just the expected challenges. Modern parenting pressures pile on extra stress. Did you just finish weaning off formula only to find a targeted ad for "toddler formula" on your social media page? Or maybe you found the perfect on-the-go yogurt snack for car rides—right before you receive unsolicited advice from a fellow parent that it should be avoided due to its sugar content. Or things are going great with solids, thank you very much—so why did your friend send you that AAP article making it seem like extended breastfeeding was something you should be prioritizing instead?

Today's parenting guidance makes it seem as if the once-fun task of feeding your toddler is actually an unsolvable puzzle. It isn't. And there is never a single answer to the questions of what and how you should feed your child. It's time to go through the basics of toddler nutrition, debunk my least favorite myths, and make eating simple and—*gasp*—*fun* again.

What Does My Toddler Need to Eat?

Let's dispel a few hard-held myths about toddler nutrition necessities. The biggest is that there is a one-size-fits-all menu you must embrace, and that your family's dietary restrictions are verboten for your little one. Incorrect. Your toddler can absolutely join you in your pescatarian, kosher, halal, vegetarian—and yes, even vegan!—diets. This remains a controversial topic in pediatrics, with doctors worried that restrictive diets will deprive little eaters of crucial macro and micronutrients. For this reason, some pediatricians still prescribe dairy—and sometimes even meat—as an absolute must. But science doesn't support that. We still don't really understand what adults are supposed to eat! As the dieting fads cycle between plant-based/vegan to all-meat/no-carbs and back again, it's clear that even scientists are often guessing. So doesn't it make more sense to figure out what molecules in food are needed for kids and build up from there?

Babies and toddlers *can* be vegan. It often takes a little more work—although these days, with more and more cuisines and brands providing vegan options, it's becoming a lot easier. Developing baby brains depend on a diet full of fat. Most vegan food is still targeted at adults, so it's likely you'll have to alter recipes, refine your shopping list, and review your takeout order so that higher-fat foods are prioritized. Skipping cow's milk will remove a major source of fat, calcium, and vitamin D for your little one. Fun fact: cow's milk convenience as a source of these ingredients (and some historical commercial lobbying) is the only reason it's framed as a mandatory component of childhood nutrition. It may take some effort to create meal plans without a one-stop-shop for these nutritional components, but it's far from impossible. There are plenty of alternative sources for nutrients your child needs.

My family didn't follow a specific diet, but I did embrace a nonprescriptive approach to what foods I offered my child during the toddler years. It was liberating, allowing me to double down on my commitment to providing variety and focusing on exploring new foods. Contrary to traditional advice (the same advice I had been giving as a pediatrician in training just years ago!) I didn't push milk. In fact, I did the opposite. My toddler loved milk, as many do, and would have chugged it all day long. But cow's milk was constipating, it can cause anemia, and my instinct told me that focusing on alternative sources of micro- and macronutrients made more sense for us. I leaned into uncertainty, remembering just how little we really understand about what makes an "ideal" diet. Encouraging food variety felt like the only reasonable choice.

Sometimes I was too committed to my mixed-up milk mission. As my daughter's milk intake ramped up, seeming to coincide perfectly with some pop science article on the purported benefits of a plant-based lifestyle, I tried to balance the equation. I was quickly foiled. She became so sensitive to my attempts at diluting her sippy cup with almond or soy milk that she learned to recognize the logos on the cartons. Pointing to the whole milk, she asked for "cow's milk" refills and cried immediately if she saw me bring out any bottle with a plant on the front. To this day, she asks for "cow's milk," lest I forget that almond, soy, oat, rice, or any nondairy substitute is simply unacceptable.

If you're stressed by the task of creating a varied customized meal plan for your family to enjoy together, help is never far away. Meeting with a pediatric nutritionist to come up with a meal plan is a great option, and you will be able to create a menu that matches your child's needs and your family's values. The truth is that almost any dietary preference can be tailored to provide kids with the nutrition they need. And if you're going the route of a more "traditional" toddler diet but still worry about nutritional requirements, it's great to chat with your pediatrician and/or pediatric nutritionist, too. Check in with experts before worrying needlessly about dietary deficiencies that the internet asserts are something to stress over (and that you should correct with a supplement or vitamin that can be "conveniently" bought with a "click here" link). A well-regulated multivitamin is fine, especially if pediatrician-approved, but in the majority of cases it's an unnecessary waste of money and energy. Unregulated supplements, as we'll review in the "Natural Disaster" chapter, carry more risk than benefit. You can ditch "immune-boosting" products and remember that a balanced diet (as best you can), promoting good sleep, and providing vaccine protection are the best ways to keep a child's immune system in tip-top shape.

What Can My Toddler Eat?

Almost anything. Besides choking hazards (like whole grapes, nuts, hard candy, unsliced hot dogs, popcorn, hunks of meat/cheese, and other uncut, hard, or chewy food), there aren't any definitive noes. The only other restriction, honey, is okay to give after a baby's first birthday. Exposing your toddler to different levels of spice, salt, and texture are all personal and cultural choices. The mantra of moderation will avoid excess. Early introduction of varied tastes will additionally help mitigate picky eating. In the end, the choice is yours. It's more than okay to make a menu that's fun to explore together as a family. Plenty of parents ditch the stress and money spent in preparing separate, so-called toddler-appropriate meals.

An important reminder: a more "baby-led weaning" style approach to family meals is great, and toddlers can 100 percent share your exact same dinner. But using more traditional "kid" food, even the prepackaged type, is totally fine as well. Pouches are convenient, and kids *like* kid food. We'll go through strategies to work through picky eating in this age group in the next chapter, and offering a shared, varied menu is a key step. It's just never all-or-none. You may have a day, week, or month where chicken nuggets and yogurt pouches constitute a large portion of your little one's dietary intake. And that's really okay.

The mantra of moderation is also key when looking at another source of parental feeding stress: so-called clean eating. It's impossible to avoid this craze, and even babies and toddlers are targeted as consumers of "nontoxic," "organic," or "natural" foods. Food science is a real and evolving field, and it's taken me years to gain an even basic understanding of what all those healthy-sounding buzzwords even mean. There's a steep learning curve, and you'll want to read up on the most up-to-date expert musings on the environmental nuances of different types of agriculture, the equity issues with "organic" farming, and why the "non-GMO" label is usually a marketing ploy. I know you'll be able to sort through it all and come up with a meal plan that matches your moral values.

Just remember to keep that healthy dose of consumer skepticism, and know that sticking to a low-stress, moderation-centered approach (especially at those cupcake-filled birthday parties) will have more health benefits than anything else. It's easy to get swept up in the idea that anything without a leafy-green label is harmful. We do, after all, live in a world where "clean" wine (which is still chock-full of toxic, liver-failure-inducing, cancer-causing alcohol) is somehow made to feel like a healthier choice than "artificial" infant formula.

But we also live in a world where environmental toxicity is very real, and a very real threat. So it's completely reasonable to try to reduce this exposure to your baby when you can—as long as the benefits of doing so are based on real science and don't create more stress than they need to. For me, this meant focusing a lot less on food labels and just doing my best to strive for variety. The reality is that the dose makes the poison, and the easiest way to minimize exposure to any toxin—be it "natural" or lab-made—is to ingest less of it. So I paid attention to broadening the culinary options available to my daughter instead of eliminating certain ingredients based on limited and questionable science.

Keep It Simple, Take 1

What's the deal with "extended breastfeeding"?

In the year 2022, when it seemed as if "pandemic parenting" couldn't bring us any new and exhausting challenges, parents across the country learned of an unimaginable new feeding dilemma: the infant-formula shortage. Our nation was ill-equipped to deal with this infant health crisis, with a slow and incomplete response that caused tremendous physical and emotional strain. And it wasn't enough to "just" leave parents unsupported, struggling to find sustenance for their babies in a society that couldn't help meet their basic needs. Instead of help, America piled on: there's no infant formula, so why don't you just breastfeed? It was a ridiculous take, devoid of any understanding of science, history, or reality. Breast-feeding is a great goal, and one that takes work. It's something parents can approach with balance by using the big-picture perspective from my first book's chapter on the topic.

The year is no longer 2022, and if you're reading this, you're likely past the point of needing infant formula. So why am I making you (and me) relive this stress? There's a rea-son, I promise. Just months into the infant-formula shortage, amid those terrible headlines asking moms to "just breast-feed," the AAP came out with an updated policy statement. It was well-intended and had an important message: parents should be supported in breastfeeding as long as they want to breastfeed. It reviewed the evidence of how breastfeeding benefits babies and added newer data showing the positive effects of breastfeeding beyond the infant years—to age two and beyond. The conclusion was that society should support breastfeeding *at least* for two years, helping parents at work and home who want to continue to provide breastmilk for their children.

While there's nothing technically wrong with any of these assertions, this AAP statement was not well received. I was among the group of parents who felt instinctively annoyed. The headlines didn't help. News sources sensationalized the statement by reducing it to "AAP says to breastfeed for two years," a grossly unfair representation. But even the full, nuanced message was ill-timed. During the formula crisis, with unscientific calls to "just breastfeed," parents were primed to receive anything as undue pressure. Even without the backdrop of a feeding crisis, our nation was already decades into a parental-support crisis. Asking for breastfeeding support beyond the first year postpartum, in a country with exactly zero days of guaranteed parental leave, was almost comical. Divorced from policy change, without tangible calls to action, the result was the same as always—a recommendation for infant health that unsupported parents would ultimately be responsible for enacting.

What should *you* do? Is extended breastfeeding right for you? Here's the simple truth: extended breastfeeding is great to do—if and only if you want to do it. The benefits of breastmilk are real, but only matter in comparison to the downside of getting that breastmilk to your baby. When nursing, pumping, or some combination of these things are no longer sustainable, you should stop. It's part of a big picture of health, and your own health and happiness contribute to that picture. Only you will know when ending your breastfeeding journey—whether it's after a few days, after a few months, or after many years—makes sense for you and your child.

Keep It Simple, Take 2

Feel free to just say no to toddler formula (unless you have a prescription from your pediatrician).

The world around us is scary and frequently overwhelming. It makes sense that today's parenting challenges are more complex than ever. Yet there are some modern worries that are so contrived, create such unnecessary anxiety, and seem to have entered the larger conversation for no other reason than to fabricate stress. I present to you: toddler formula.

All effective advertising works by convincing us that something is missing. You can't sell something without highlighting a deficiency, then promising that a product is the secret to filling that void. It's a frequently exaggerated void, and it's always good to take a step back before embracing consumerist solutions. Chances are that whatever magic bullet is marketed your way isn't strictly necessary. Your parenting isn't broken, no need to fix it. Sometimes, however, a void isn't exaggerated—it's simply made up.

Toddler formulas are a prime example of something you just do not need—at least, not without your pediatrician's medical recommendation. Some degree of picky eating in the toddler years is the norm, not the exception (stay tuned for lots more in the next chapter). But even with fussy feeding habits, the vast majority of children meet all their nutritional needs through regular food and drink. Absent a medical or behavioral issue, a toddler who is growing well, is offered a variety of nutrient-rich foods, and is allowed to eat (or not) when they're hungry (or not), will be able to provide themselves with the nutrition they require.

Contrary to insidious marketing, there is no evidence of widespread deficiency of macro- or micronutrients in this age group. This makes toddler formula at best a waste of money and energy. However, replacing ongoing culinary exploration and varied food exposure with an unnecessary nutritional shake has developmental consequences. We know that consuming solid food plays a crucial role in fine motor and sensory development. It is also a mainstay of social development, facilitating family meals, and allowing you to take the steps we'll review in the next chapter to model and strengthen a healthy, adventurous relationship with food.

Ironically, I use toddler formulas all the time. I'm a pediatrician at a large academic children's hospital, which means I care for a *ton* of patients with complex medical issues. Many of my patients require these supplements as part or all of their nutritional intake. I also care for children whose picky eating is more than just picky eating. ARFID (avoidant restrictive food intake disorder), autism spectrum disorder, or medical/behavioral conditions can lead to malnourishment if we don't prescribe these formulas. It's my appreciation of advances in supplemental nutrition that makes me so wary of its widespread use. It's the direct-to-parent marketing, where companies suggest that all toddlers must incorporate formula into their diets, that is so deeply frustrating. These corporations may be turning their eyes to a wider market, but it's best to keep a discussion of toddler formula where it belongs—between you and your pediatrician, as part of a larger conversation about your child's health and nutrition.

THE BOTTOM LINE

5 out of 5 Pediatrician Parents Agree

1. Toddlers can follow whatever diet fits your family's personal, ethical, and cultural preference. Worry less about specific food ingredients and instead embrace variety, paying attention to the macro- and micronutrients your child needs. A pediatric nutritionist is a great resource, whether or not your family has dietary restrictions.

2. Cow's milk is not mandatory. There are plenty of alternative sources to the nutrients it (conveniently) provides.

3. Your toddler can eat anything that isn't a choking hazard. I like offering "adult" food to kids as much as your lifestyle allows, prioritizing family meals and a positive relationship with food. Pouches, nuggets, and "kids meals" are beloved and convenient, okay to give, but not mandatory.

4. If you can, stay somewhat flexible with food, especially in social situations and outside the home. Encouraging a fun relationship with eating helps avoid pathologizing "unhealthy" or "artificial" food and makes moderation easier for your child later on. Letting your child celebrate with peers (think birthday cupcakes and ice cream parties) without restriction reaps social and emotional rewards that should be balanced against your personal food preferences.

5. "Clean eating" is a fad. Food science is real and complex, but claims of "nontoxic," or "natural" are reductive and unhelpful. "Organic" doesn't always mean healthier or more environmentally friendly.

6. There's no need for toddler formula unless there's a medical reason—i.e., your pediatrician prescribes it. It's, at best, a waste of money and, at worst, interferes with food exploration and makes picky-eating habits harder to work on.

7. Extended breastfeeding (giving breastmilk beyond one year) is great and should be supported by society. It's only great for you, however, if it's great for you. Asking society to support parents isn't the same as asking you to change your breastfeeding goals. You should still wean off breastfeeding whenever is best for your family.

CHAPTER 7

PICKY EATING

Preventing Pathologically Picky Eating When You Can and How to Deal With It When You Can't

I was unintentionally—and I like to think adorably—a pretentious child when it came to eating. I wanted nothing more than to be offered a world of culinary exploration. At the age of five, I fearlessly ordered foie gras off the menu—and loved it. My restaurant tantrums were reserved for times when the waiter, understandably, brought me the kid's menu, which I found deeply offensive. (Oh, how I wish the delicious and cost-effective kids' menu were still available to me now!) Most of the kids in my family were the same way—miniature gourmands demanding the standard prix fixe meal with their crayons and placemats.

Growing up among precocious eaters made me less equipped than many parents when it came to dealing with my own child's picky eating. As my daughter entered the toddler years, I was basking in the success of a modified baby-led weaning approach. She loved it, and it was a joyful parenting "win" to be able to share saag paneer for lunch and arroz con pollo for dinner. Alas, it seemed as if I flew too close to the sun. At fifteen months, as the food rejections escalated from reasonable (kale salad? Pass) to absurd (did you know that there's a "wrong" color of macaroni and cheese?), I wondered how I would ever get my daughter to try new foods again.

It's no secret that the toddler years can be a challenging time to optimize nutrition. It's the rare toddler who doesn't go through picky-eating phases, and even the best baby-led weaning plans can go awry when those toddler food preferences kick in. Don't worry. I made it through, and so will you. This chapter will walk you through the basics of toddler food fussiness and share the hard-earned lessons I learned so that your experience can be as healthy and low-stress as possible.

What Is Picky Eating? Is It Normal?

It would be nice to have a clear definition of "picky eating" before we dive into the topic. Alas, it's hard to find a single set of criteria that scientists use when studying picky eating, and nonscientific sources use even more widely variable, looser definitions. Many, but not all, definitions require that eating is only "picky" when it leads to inadequate intake. We all seem to agree that being "picky" means rejecting a significant number of foods offered. Scientists also agree that as infants transition into the toddler years, some degree of "neophobia"—the rejection of new foods—is normal.

Picky eating is common, but it's hard to say just how common it is. Some studies estimate the prevalence of picky eating in toddlers to be as high as 50 percent. But definitions are so variable that, depending on what you consider "picky," the real number could be much higher or lower than this. What we can say for sure is that picky eating— even the kind that parents feel is excessive—is extremely common.

The good thing about picky eating during the toddler years is that it tends to stay in the toddler years. Most kids' pickiness improves, especially if caretakers set the stage for food exploration and a positive relationship with food. Even pickiness that parents perceive as pathological tends to go away on its own.

When Is It a Problem?

Picky eating that doesn't meet specific criteria for pathology (causing medical effects) isn't a problem if it's not a problem. Meaning, if it's not leading to psychosocial issues, interfering with school or activities, or functionally making your life impossible, it's okay to just watch and wait.

There's more than common sense and clinical experience behind this approach. We also have data. There are studies that show kids who are "picky" eaters take in the same number of calories as their more adventurous counterparts. The same studies are also generally reassuring about macro- and micronutrient intake, which doesn't seem to be affected in meaningful ways by "pickiness." What's more, this is true even when selective eating persists into later years. Some research suggests zinc and iron can decrease, but it's unclear how this plays out in the real world, especially since these minerals are frequently low in kids to begin with. It's a good reminder to talk to your pediatrician if you have any concerns. In the majority of cases, if your child is growing, a multivitamin (or, more likely, not!) is all you'll need to stay on track.

That's all to say, picky eating is rarely a problem. But cases when picky eating is clearly pathological do exist. I see a disproportionate number of these cases as a hospital pediatrician. It's my job to find the root cause and give families individualized treatment. The differential diagnosis for picky eating—the kind that leads to serious nutritional deficiency, poor growth, and often comes alongside other symptoms— is broad. We'd need a medical school lecture series just to scratch the surface of potential causes: sensory processing disorders (which can be linked to autism spectrum disorders); gastrointestinal or inflammatory conditions; infections; autoimmune disease; and many others. It's my job as a doctor to take a good history, decide which tests make sense, and create a game plan. That's *not* your job, so there's no need to become an expert on the pediatric gastrointestinal and metabolic systems. Just know that not eating enough food can be a part of a variety of fixable medical and behavioral disorders.

There are some red flags that signal a medical issue is more likely, such as pain with eating, vomiting, or other signs of underlying inflammation (fevers, diarrhea, rashes, weight loss). There are also rare cases where picky eating itself is pathological, meaning a child's food refusal is so severe that growth and nutritional problems develop. This is known as avoidant restrictive food intake disorder (ARFID), a condition with specific clinical criteria that I've treated many times as a hospital pediatrician. I mention this particular diagnosis to highlight an important point: pathological picky eating is a medical diagnosis. If all other potential causes of food avoidance have been ruled out, but your child still isn't eating enough to grow and thrive, we can still help. ARFID is treatable, and a prime example of when significant psycho-social or medical damage from picky eating means it's not just picky eating—it's pathological, and it's time to get help.

Anything outside of this medical zone of pathological picky eating lands you in the typical toddler eating zone—and if you're still not quite sure, ask your pediatrician! Setting expectations is key. Yes, you may find yourself raising the rare, pretentious toddler (like yours truly) who demands pâtè and caviar. But it's far more likely you'll find yourself dealing with fussy feeding habits and frequent food refusal. Instead of fighting against fate, take time to review these strategies. Embracing these techniques will help you deal, and help your toddler create the best relationship with food possible—the most important goal and best way to promote adventurous eating in the future.

That's a Lot of What Not to Do. But What Can You Do to Cope with Your Toddler's Feeding Fuss?

1. *Rest on your "BLW" laurels and keep it going—or try it for the first time!*

As I detailed in *Parent Like a Pediatrician,* I love baby-led weaning in large part because it sets the stage for food exploration and variety. As a quick recap, the principle of a BLW-style approach is simple: ditch purees as much as possible and focus on finger foods, letting your infant decide what they want to explore and when. Baby-led weaning gives infants the chance early on—when tastes are developing—to experience a rich and varied diet. Countless studies on infant feeding prove that tiny babies will try anything. If you've adopted some of these baby-led strategies, bask in the culinary curriculum you've provided and keep the trend of food exploration going. If you did a more traditional introduction to solids, that's okay, too! It's never too late to broaden your child's palate. Feel free to start sharing the exact same, varied menu you put on your own plate, letting your little one place whatever they want to try (other than the choking hazards we reviewed in chapter 6) in their mouth and develop gustatory, oromotor, and social skills.

2. *Prioritize social meals.*

Focusing on social meals is one of my favorite strategies. I'm a big fan of family dinners, trying to offer the same (or similar) food for the whole family. My aim has always been to put whatever food I'm offering my daughter on her plate and emphasize that she only has to try what she wants to.

Pouring your energy into family eating behavior is one of the most important evidence-based interventions. Studies show that balanced eating by parents is a predictor of less picky eating in their children later on. Having a single family menu makes mealtime less stressful; shared meals minimize prep time, and consolidating dinnertime into a single session will restore some precious time that you'd otherwise be spending on micromanaging a toddler meal. When the focus is on an enjoyable family dining experience, eating becomes fun, not a chore.

An important caveat: relaxed eating with whatever dietary preferences your family decides on, is only healthy if you share nutritious foods. Studies consistently show that how healthy a family eats at home is the best way to predict how healthy a kid will be. It's not about restrictions. Simply having nutritious options available and providing a varied menu is all you need. It's what sets the stage for years of good eating, appropriate weight gain, and overall well-being.

Another important caveat: when I say "prioritize social meals" the key word is *prioritize,* meaning a family meal with a single menu isn't achievable one hundred percent of the time. And how strongly or consistently you prioritize this goal will vary as well. I've personally cycled through plenty of phases—sometimes weeks or more—where a modified toddler menu was all I had time to prepare. Even more frequently, I lack the motivation needed to enforce any all-ages menu and instead lean into a cycle of mac-and-cheese/hot dogs/pizza bites dinners because it's the easiest path for everyone. I know that pauses in the adventurous eating education I'm providing aren't forever and won't lead to permanent harm. And even imperfect adherence to a family meal plan on your part reaps benefits primarily by modeling the attitudes and behaviors you want your child to develop *over time*. In the short term, the result may be the same limited toddler intake, regardless of whether you offer them a five-course menu next to the chicken nuggets they (exclusively) devour. So be flexible, be patient, and remember perfect is the enemy of good when it comes to toddler food variety.

3. Remember: you control what you offer, not what they eat.

Repeat after me: you control what foods, and when, you offer food to your child. They control if they eat, and how much. It's the new mantra of experts in pediatric feeding. If there's only one thing you take from this chapter, let it be this immutable, liberating truth.

There's no amount of social meals, BLW, or commitment to food exploration that can override your child's willpower. Promoting adventurous eating from the very first bite doesn't guarantee your toddler won't binge on yogurt pouches and french fries for a week at a time. But the combination of some sort of modified/extended baby-led weaning, offering varied and healthy choices, and keeping the stress out of mealtime will prevent most picky eating from becoming pathologic.

Letting go is an evidence-based strategy. Studies show that pressuring children to eat makes pickiness worse—and of course is a source of counterproductive stress. When the temptation to count the number of foods your child will eat arises, or you find yourself "encouraging" veggie intake to no avail, take a step back. Put whatever you want on your child's plate, and see what happens. If they leave half their meal untouched (surprise, it's mostly broccoli that remains!) that's okay. If they're still hungry, they'll ask for more food, and you'll pour your energy into choosing their next option (how about some more of that yummy lasagna they were so brave to try?) instead of frustrating everyone with a low-yield battle to embrace bitter vegetables.

I wouldn't have believed any of this if I hadn't tried it myself—successfully. I've also helped countless parents embrace a similarly chill approach with equally rave reviews. It wasn't easy to dive so deeply into a laissez-faire, food-neutral mindset. As parents, we are hardwired to worry about what our kids eat! And with a barrage of endless, conflicting information on what constitutes optimal nutrition and eating behavior, it's hard not to feel overwhelmed. But it *can* be simple. Barring medical or behavioral issues, you can trust your toddler to autoregulate their intake. You can decide that all the food you offer is great, in moderation. You can serve dessert at the same time as dinner (yes, I absolutely do this!), and let them decide what they want to eat first. You can remind them that there's still chicken and avocado on their plate after they undoubtedly eat the cookies there first and cry for more. You can focus on shopping, cooking, ordering takeout, making smiley-face fruit plates and reject the stress of monitoring their intake. If you respect your child's hunger cues—and teach them to respect their own—they will consume the amount of food that is exactly right for their body.

4. Nothing is forever.

Toddlers don't have "tastes"; they just have moods. There's no way to know what a toddler will want to eat on any given day, at any given meal, at any given second. So just keep trying, and the rest will be what it may be. It's why I try to avoid labeling foods as ones that my daughter "likes" or "dislikes." Whenever possible, I talk about whether a food is one she's tried before or not, and if she would like to try it now or reconsider later.

5. Don't force it.

If you have access to nutrient-rich foods, and offer them to your child, you're halfway to completing your parental feeding duties. The only other, equally crucial task is to promote a fun and healthy relationship with food. I can't stress enough how important it is to set the stage for a positive eating experience early on in life. As a hospital pediatrician, I've treated more than my fair share of toddlers who can't gain weight—and even need feeding tubes—because they simply refuse to eat. It's called an oral aversion, and usually happens when kids were sick early on and developed bad associations with being forced to eat. It's an extreme that gives credence to a commonsense philosophy: forcing a kid to eat can have long-term consequences.

6. *Keep it loose where you can.*

You can rest assured that allowing your toddler to have a slice of cake at a birthday party won't undo all the hard-earned benefits of a healthy at-home diet. In fact, steering away from overly stringent dietary rules is one of the most important ingredients to providing your little one with a balanced relationship with food. And what the science consistently shows us is that it's just as important—if not more important—to focus on how you frame access to sweets, treats, and assorted processed goodies as it is to make sure they aren't consumed in excess.

The mantra of moderation is a great way to make sure that eating is as nourishing to the body and mind as possible, and that it stays that way. Only you will know what the ideal menu looks like for your family, based on whatever combination of personal, ethical, religious, and cultural principles matter most to you. And only you will know how strictly you want to extend those preferences to when your child is outside of the home. So you'll want to make sure that you've done the right amount of reflection—and research—to help you decide what food convictions you hold, and why they are meaningful to you.

THE BOTTOM LINE

5 out of 5 Pediatrician Parents Agree

1. "Picky"-eating habits during the toddler years are the norm, not the exception. Even when fussy food habits seem excessive, they rarely lead to nutritional problems and usually get better on its own. When in doubt, your pediatrician will help you decide if a medical or behavioral condition needs to be diagnosed and addressed.

2. In the vast majority of cases, taking a low-stress approach is the way to go. Picky eating is only a "problem" when it is related to medical issues, has psychological effects, or interferes with social and daily life activities.

3. Putting excessive pressure on eating certain types or amounts of food often makes picky eating worse. There are even extreme cases where eating anxiety can lead to pathological restrictions in intake. If your pediatrician agrees that your toddler's nutrition is on track, it's best to stay patient and hands-off.

4. While you wait, you can use mealtime strategies that promote a positive relationship with food. The most important technique is based on the fact that your child, if there's no medical or psychological problem, will autoregulate hunger. This means that you control what you offer, they control what they eat. Telling toddlers to "clean your plate" is so 1996.

5. Stay adventurous and keep it social. Family meals, snacks with friends, exploring different cuisines are all ways to keep feeding fun and model trying new things.

6. Toddlers don't have "tastes"; they just have "moods." I avoid "like" and "dislike" and instead frame foods as those we want to try now, or those we'll consider again later.

7. Moderation is king. Worry less about specific foods, ingredients, and portion size. Offer a varied menu, minimizing labels of "healthy" and "unhealthy," and adding in sweets wherever and whenever feels right to you. Birthday cupcakes, ice cream at the park, or even routine dessert at home (served in our house on the same plate as dinner!) help take sugary treats off a pedestal.

CHAPTER 8

TODDLER SLEEP-SCHEDULE UPDATES

Breaking Down Myth versus Fact About Your Child's Evolving Nap and Bedtime Needs

The toddler years mark so many transitions, many of which we've spent the past chapters reviewing. Another major milestone? Just how awake and alert your little one has become. Your child has evolved from a creature who slept most of the day into an active, high-energy human. Congratulations!

As energetic as your child has become, they still need a lot of rest. There's so much growing to do! But how much rest is the right amount? Toddlers aren't ready to ditch naps altogether, but how many do they need? All the other kids at daycare seem to take longer naps—is that okay? Or, some parents wonder instead, why does everyone else in your child's playgroup seem to take shorter naps? Or nap more often? Are these variations really normal? Somehow, despite best intentions, many parents find themselves doubting their toddlers' (almost certainly) healthy sleep habits just as much as they did in infancy.

Naptime worries are a needless source of parental angst in the toddler years. Let's update our approach to sleep schedules, making sure everyone can stress less and get the rest they deserve.

General Toddler Sleep Needs

Pediatricians understand much of the complex neuroscience of sleep in children, countless sleep disorders, the general amount of sleep a child needs, and overall trends in napping. We often explain these to parents in a quick one-page handout. At toddler checkups, these handouts will state that according to the latest AAP consensus, children aged one to five years average a total of ten to fourteen hours of sleep per day. How this is divided is variable. In general, naps become less frequent during the toddler years, often going from three times per day to as little as once daily. At what point kids "should" drop their nap is still up for debate. Some kids have trouble sleeping during the day by their second birthday, but many will do well with a scheduled nap through kindergarten.

The frustrating reality is that when it comes to deciding what the ideal amount of toddler sleep is, science doesn't have a numeric answer. Yes, there are plenty of studies that show sleep deprivation can cause problems. Children who get lower quality sleep, or sleep much less than the typical amount, may have developmental and cognitive issues. Whether this is a direct result or not is hard to say. Ethically, no studies on sleep deprivation in children are controlled clinical trials (we would never force children to stay awake just to see how this affects them). Poor sleep is often a marker of other life stressors, including other health conditions, and the links we find are associations. But from what we know about the importance of sleep in all humans, it's a good bet that not letting kids meet their sleep needs will have consequences.

Let's reread that last sentence, because the key point of this statement often gets overlooked. It's not about how much sleep your kid gets compared to the rest of the population. It's about how much sleep your kid gets compared to *their specific needs*. There are healthy, happy toddlers who get fewer than ten hours of sleep each day. There are also tired toddlers who get fourteen hours of sleep but could still use another nap. Sleep norms are different for each child, each family, each culture. Anyone pitching a one-size-fits-all approach to your kid's sleep habits is missing the bigger picture.

Averages are averages, an elusive truth that leads to needless parenting stress. As we explored in our nutrition and picky-eating chapters, the reality is that just like children know how to eat, they also know how to sleep. We've been doing a pretty bad job of giving toddlers credit for the (relatively few) things they are in fact able to do expertly. Regulating their own sleep needs—and letting you know if you're doing an okay job of letting them meet these needs— is something they actually are awesome at doing.

I repeat: like infants, toddlers are born to autoregulate sleep. If you give them adequate stimulation when awake, let them sleep when tired, and don't consistently force them to stay up when they'd rather be snoozing, there's no biological concern that they will be sleep-deprived (or somehow over-rested). And remember, who's driving the ship is key. There's a big difference between a toddler who is constantly woken up from naps to fit an overstuffed schedule of activities and a toddler who wakes up on their own from short naps because that's what their body craves.

A quick caveat—the truism of sleep autoregulation as an innate human ability doesn't mean that sleep issues aren't real. Just like adults, children can have issues falling and staying asleep—which we will cover in detail in the next chapter. In these situations, troubleshooting sleep habits and medical/behavioral challenges is a necessary task. But this isn't the same as worrying something is "wrong" with your toddler when an arbitrary, universal sleep schedule doesn't work for them.

Nap Schedules—What's the Deal?

There's no evidence to support that kids on firm nap schedules are somehow healthier than those whose naptimes are more flexible. Think about it: What are the chances that, over the course of human history, normal development was dependent on a fixed sleep schedule? It's exceedingly more likely that our species, instead, evolved under circumstances where parents let babies and toddlers sleep at will—or whenever it fit into an already busy schedule of survival. A strict napping routine is indeed a modern, made-up worry. But we also happen to live in a modern world. Even the most easygoing caretakers need some structure to build their day around. Whether it's being cared for by a nanny, at daycare, or at home with Mom or Dad, it's the rare situation where some basic naptime plan isn't helpful. So while there may be no developmental need for your child to have a stringent nap schedule, there are definitely benefits to caretakers creating some discrete sleep times.

Even though I'm totally on board with embracing a sleep schedule, the principle of adaptability (to life's circumstances and your child's evolving needs) reigns supreme. Instead of pledging allegiance to the one-size-fits-all nap guide you saw online, try to follow these guidelines:

1. You're the expert in your child's sleep needs.

As a parent, you're the boss of your family and the expert in your child's needs. Full stop. This means that you are the best person to decide when the task of creating a sleep schedule is worthwhile for the structure it provides. And it also means that you know better than anyone else how much sleep they require.

I mean it. You don't need a PhD in the neuroscience of sleep to figure out if your kid is getting enough sleep or not. Those nap charts—and check-ins with your pediatrician—are a great start. But remember, you've been watching your child sleep their whole life! You know their evolving sleep trends, the cues that they're tired, the happy, alert play signaling a nap well-taken. You'll absolutely be able to use these patterns, combined with the reality of your own day-to-day routine, to create a general sleep schedule that fits everyone's needs.

Meeting your child's sleep needs doesn't necessarily mean fitting their exact, "natural" sleep schedule to a tee. Even when external factors alter their innate sleep patterns, chances are they'll be able to adapt. When my daughter started daycare, I panicked that the shorter, less frequent nap schedule would turn her into a sleep-deprived baby zombie. But it absolutely worked out. Depending on her nap-needs de jour, she was able to take a rest in the "cozy corner," sleep during our commute (thanks, New York City rush-hour traffic!), or doze at home on the couch before dinner. When biology and reality aren't perfectly aligned, check in on your child before jumping straight to worry. You can trust yourself to assess their restedness and make changes if your routine really isn't working.

If you still find yourself stressing over how much sleep your toddler is getting, remember that a quick call to your pediatrician will outsource the worry and sort through things in no time. And if your child is "lethargic," seems impossible to wake up, or has any change in activity that just doesn't seem right, definitely let us know! Serious problems are rare—the most likely explanation is an undetected virus that needs some extra snuggles—but as always, there's no need to triage on your own.

2. Stay flexible—as much as you can, at least.

Ever had a day so exciting that you couldn't fall asleep for hours? What about an exhausting day that had you passed out on the couch before dinner?

Kids, like every adult I've ever met, would answer yes to these questions if they could. There will be plenty of times when your toddler, no matter how easily they go down for a typical nap, is just not able to sleep according to their usual schedule. And that's okay. Expect to have the (at least) occasional "off" day, whether it's because your kid was too tired to stick to their routine, because you had to adjust it for a special event, or simply because your childcare fell through and you just couldn't pull your act together at home. When "off" days become patterns, it's often because there's a nap-time transition point approaching. Is your child tired all the time and can't make it to their next nap? Maybe a nap was dropped a little too soon. Consistently fighting that morning nap no matter what you do? Could be time to consolidate and shift the schedule. Keeping attuned to their cues, and responding to the patterns you see, will assure that they get the necessary amount of rest to grow and thrive.

3. Don't forget about bedtime!

An additional pro tip: Being tired really is the enemy of sleep. It's why so many parents find that the solution to super-early morning awakenings or naptime struggles is actually to push bedtime even earlier. I'm a huge fan of this as well, with plenty of personal and professional success stories. Does that mean there's anything inherently "wrong" with raising your kid as a night owl? No, and there are absolutely parents who favor a later bedtime, have children who still sleep through the night, with the whole family still staying well rested.

Getting good rest—whatever that looks like for your kid—is the key to a successful sleep schedule. It's why I do agree that "sleep begets sleep," however your little one interprets that rule. Just like most toddlers do better with a bedtime routine that starts earlier (usually when they're less tired), they often do better with an uninterrupted afternoon nap. So while I don't think it's fair to say you should "never wake a sleeping baby," we can definitely dispel the myth that allowing a child to nap too late will disrupt bedtime. I can personally attest to an extreme example of this not being true, with my daughter frequently napping up until just an hour before bedtime—and still going to bed as easily (and sleeping as long) as usual. Letting little ones nap as much as their bodies crave tends to be more conducive to a good bedtime than waking them up after a certain amount of time. As a rule, getting a good night's sleep has more to do with how parents put their kids to sleep and much less with when the children's naps end (check out those bedtime routines we'll review in our "Sleep Regression" chapter). Stay attuned to the patterns you see and embrace a whole lot of trial and error. I promise you'll be able to find a schedule that works for you, recognizing the strategies that actually improve your little one's restfulness.

THE BOTTOM LINE

5 out of 5 Pediatrician Parents Agree

1. Toddlers get an *average* of ten to fourteen hours of sleep per day. Most kids do best with a daytime nap (or more) during this age group, but how their bodies like to divide sleep throughout the day is highly variable.

2. Toddlers, like all humans, need high-quality sleep. But this doesn't mean they need to sleep as long or as frequently as other children; it means they need to meet their *own* sleep needs.

3. Humans are born to autoregulate sleep, and toddlers are humans. If given enough opportunity to sleep—after troubleshooting any medical and/or behavioral challenges that arise—toddlers will get the amount of sleep that's right for them.

4. There's no biological "need" for a formal nap schedule. However, some sort of sleep routine makes daily living easier for toddlers and caretakers in most situations.

5. You're the expert in your child's sleep needs, making you the expert in creating your child's sleep schedule. There will be external factors that help shape your plan (daycare, nannies, playgroups, and more), so don't worry if naptime isn't perfectly aligned with what your child does in the wild. Focus instead on how your child is adapting to these external routines and trust yourself to make changes if things aren't working.

6. Stay flexible, as much as you can. There are plenty of times where an activity is important enough to make a rescheduled naptime worthwhile. It's also common for toddlers to have "off days," making day-to-day flexibility and focusing more on patterns the way to go.

7. Don't forget about bedtime! Being tired is the enemy of sleep. When naptime issues arise, doubling down on bedtime routines is often the best remedy.

CHAPTER 9

THE DREADED TODDLER SLEEP REGRESSION

Troubleshooting Your Little One's Sleep Issues So You Can All Get the Best Rest Possible

F inally. Your little one is sleeping through the night (or close to it). After a hard-fought battle with sleep training, or just patient waiting, your baby learned how to dream in their crib long enough for you to actually get a good night's rest. You're on top of the world, simply crushing parenting.

This was exactly how I felt at the one-year mark. And this is exactly what made the appearance of toddler sleep issues so painful. It felt as if I had flown too close to the sun, basked a little too warmly in the light of a full night's sleep, and crashed suddenly into the nightmare of sleep regressions. In our case, it was the first daycare-sponsored virus that plunged our enviable routine back into the realm of multiple overnight awakenings. Later on, life transitions, illnesses, and growth spurts continued to challenge our reestablished sleep schedule. Each regression was exhausting, overwhelming, and disappointing.

Each time, though, I found ways to make things easier, and to get through it a little more quickly. Toddler sleep regressions are extremely common, and general toddler sleep struggles are universal. Let's break down the basics of toddler sleep issues and learn some strategies for how to get through them as painlessly as possible.

Sleep Regressions 101

Even if your toddler is getting enough rest overall, it's likely you'll encounter some sleep challenges at some point. In fact, about a third of parents report dealing with significant sleep issues during the toddler years, and many more express a desire to optimize their child's sleep. Sleep regressions—often defined by more frequent night awakenings—are one of the most common and frustrating issues that parents cite. We have lots of data from around the world showing that while overnight awakenings decrease in frequency by age one, they are still something the majority of toddlers (74 percent in a recent, large study) will experience—at least from time to time. Another type of "regression," fighting bedtime, is also common, and a frequent source of parental stress. I promise you aren't alone. In a recent study, researchers looked at an "Ask the Expert" social media thread that had 1,287 questions about toddler sleep. Most of these questions—85 percent—were about night awakenings, sleep schedules, and bedtime problems.

Why do toddlers seem to suddenly forget how to sleep? There's no single answer. Backtracking in sleep routines often happens when toddlers don't feel well, both physically and emotionally. Viruses are a common reason for overnight awakenings, as are life transitions and social stressors. Sometimes, there's no clear trigger. Scientists hypothesize that periods of rapid growth can disrupt established sleep routines, or that normal variation in sleep patterns (which evolve with age) are to blame.

Sleep Regression Strategies—a.k.a. That's a Nice Explanation but How Do I Deal?

Sleep struggles are common, stressful, and unpredictable. If and when the dreaded toddler sleep regression finds its way into your home, you can use the following principles and strategies to make it through.

1. Everyone's different.

It's easy, even years into the sleep troubleshooting game, to get swept up in the hype. I still find conflicting, black-and-white guidance on the topic of toddler sleep every day on my social media feed—even when I'm not seeking it out. When less scrupulous sleep trainers continue to sell you on the myth that a certain amount of uninterrupted sleep, in a certain setting, with a certain bedtime routine is the best for every kid, you can remember this can't be true. Yes, there are certainly ways to optimize quality sleep and create the sleep routine that works best for your family. But there's no evidence that a particular location for sleeping, or a particular age for sleeping through the night without getting up and seeking parents, is inherently best for your child.

On the opposite end of the spectrum from rigid sleep training mandates, you will find strict "attachment parenting" guides that purport that anything other than indefinite bed sharing is child abuse. Plenty of sources incorrectly assert that the only way to achieve "biologically normal" sleep for your child is to literally share a bed with them up to and even through the teenage years! Extremes are never the answer. Experts agree that the "best" sleep for your kid depends on so many factors. Not only are sleep needs different for each person, but there are cultural, geographical, and individual differences in what we define as normal sleep. Your child is the expert in their own sleep, and there are plenty of ways to help them—and you—reach that delicious goal of getting high-quality, minimally uninterrupted rest.

When it comes to sleep regressions, this principle is specifically freeing and particularly salient. If, how, and when you decide to troubleshoot bedtime issues and over-night awakenings will depend on if there's even an issue to troubleshoot. If you're like me, any sleep interruption is automatically a problem, and my threshold to intervene is much lower than a parent with different sleep practices and preferences. Plenty of others are more than fine letting their littles crawl into bed for periods of time, short and long. Yes, it might be more challenging (but not impossible) to reverse sleep routines later on, but there's no law saying you can't snuggle with your toddler in the middle of the night if that fits your style. And if you decide that promoting independent sleep from an early age is super important (like I did!), don't let a single online shamer make you feel that encouraging your kid to sleep in their own room is harmful.

2. It's all connected!

If you decide to intervene when your child keeps waking up in the middle of the night, it can be easy to focus only on the perceived problem at hand. The most common example I see (and have lived through) is when overnight awakenings steal the spotlight. It's tempting to pour all of our (beyond-exhausted, middle-of-the-night) energy into getting your toddler back to sleep on their own. But just like with infant sleep training, many find that shifting that energy back to bedtime actually reaps more benefits.

Bedtime issues, overnight awakenings, and sleep struggles in general are all intricately interconnected. And conveniently enough, focusing on just one element (namely, bedtime) seems to be the most evidence-based strategy to fixing many different areas of sleep. It makes sense physiologically. As I've said, being tired is the enemy of sleep for toddlers just as it is for infants. Optimizing bedtime leads to better sleep, staving off issues later in the night. And as you may remember from infant sleep training, overnight awakenings are universal—for infants, children, and adults alike. We all wake up frequently throughout the night, and most of us decide we are tired enough (and feel safe enough) to fall back asleep where we are. When babies and kids are scared, uncomfortable, overstimulated, or even overtired, they seek your help in feeling comfortable enough to fall back asleep. It's something they *can* learn to do on their own. It's why in Ferber-esque sleep training techniques, there's often no need to interfere in overnight awakenings. Focusing on teaching kids how to fall asleep on their own at bedtime eventually translates to being able to fall back asleep when they wake up in the middle of the night.

There's emerging evidence proving the pediatrician-approved principle of focusing on bedtime routines when troubleshooting any sleep issue. Some of the highest quality studies on toddler sleep that we have available show that in households where bedtime routines are consistent and prioritized, overall sleep is improved. In the end, if you double down on bedtime routines, fine-tune sleep hygiene measures (no screens near bedtime, for example), and even redo a mini Ferber-style bedtime sleep training if bedtime struggles are an issue, you will likely see all different types of sleep regressions fade away.

3. It's okay to wait.

Sometimes there's an identifiable trigger for your little one's sleep regression. Any life transition frequently manifests in sleep issues, and in an ever-changing world, there's likely some stressor that is at least contributing to, if not underlying, your toddler's new sleep behavior. Facing back-to-back viral illnesses that make overnight snuggles logical and necessary? New sibling, new move, new school, new anything? There's a good chance that your child's sleep regression comes at a time of real stress for everyone. And there's a good chance that "indulging" overnight awakenings is less exhausting, at least for a few days (or weeks, or even months), than striving to return to independent sleep as quickly as possible.

4. Try a bedtime pass.

When the dust settles, and you decide that you can't wait much longer to get your little one back to their wake-free overnight sleep routine, there are options. Definitely keep optimizing that bedtime routine (with or without a modified reprise of your infant sleep training techniques) to get the most bang for your sleep-troubleshooting buck. If there's any suspicion of a medical or more serious emotional problem (I'll go through a few common ones soon), absolutely check in with your pediatrician. After this, my favorite intervention is a "bedtime pass."

It's an easy, commonsense tool that I learned from the expert pediatrician parents when I was training as a resident. At the beginning of the night, you'll give your toddler some sort of "ticket" that lets them come into your bed overnight should the need arise. No shame or judgment—you understand that it's something they may still want to do for a bit! If they do, they'll give you their "pass" before climbing into your bed. If they don't, though, and have their pass in the morning, they get a prize. I'm a fan of activity-based prizes when possible (like going to a favorite destination together), but old-fashioned toy prizes do the trick, too. This technique clearly works best at older developmental stages, and I see the most success after age two, when kids understand the concept of delayed gratification at least a little bit. It's easier when they're sleeping in a bed and can walk themselves into your room, but you can modify it for crib sleepers and grab the token from their bedside when you come to pick them up.

If this approach isn't feasible at all, I've seen some parents bring their (usually gradual) sleep training techniques into the overnight hours, letting their toddlers cry for various intervals before going to pick them up. With my overnight exhaustion approaching delirium, this wouldn't have been a good option for me. And the truth is that for most kids, waiting just a few extra days while channeling all efforts into bedtime strategies solves the issue completely.

Sleepwalking, Night Terrors, Obstructive Sleep Apnea, and More

Sleep regressions are normal, a standard toddler parent rite of passage. But there are times where there's a medical sleep problem underlying your sleep woes—or at least contributing to them. It's never your job to diagnose or treat on your own, so you'll be booking an appointment with your pediatrician if there's any concern! Let's review some of the more common toddler sleep disorders so you'll be prepared if they arise (and have a head start for your pediatrician visit).

1. OSA/snoring

What is it?

When we talk about snoring in kids, there are a few different diagnoses we can give. The two you're most likely to come across are primary snoring and sleep apnea. Primary snoring just means a kid snores but doesn't stop breathing or have their blood oxygen level drop. Snoring can also be related to a condition called obstructive sleep apnea (OSA). With OSA, something happens to block the passage of air in and out of the upper airway. With this diagnosis, there are pauses in breathing (apneas) and brief periods of low oxygen levels in the blood.

What causes it?

There are lots of reasons kids can snore—allergies, cold viruses, their lung and airway anatomy. If it's primary snoring, there's not much to do other than treat any underlying causes if they need to be treated. Your pediatrician will want to rule out OSA, though, since they are so closely related. OSA also has a lot of possible causes. Some of the conditions that your pediatrician will look into are large adenoids and tonsils, upper airway issues, and facial anatomical differences, just to name a few.

How common is it?

As you may have guessed, snoring is more common than OSA. Studies estimate that between 10 and 12 percent of children snore on a routine basis. OSA is relatively rare in children, especially compared to adults: around 1 to 3 percent of children get diagnosed with this condition.

What are the symptoms?

Primary snoring is generally asymptomatic besides the obvious symptom: snoring. When sleep apnea is the issue, there are frequently (but not always) other symptoms that signal this issue. During the night parents may observe snoring, restless sleep, sudden episodes of waking up, waking up gasping for air or choking, bed wetting, excessive sweating, and even sleepwalking. As a result of low-quality sleep, there can also be daytime symptoms—usually sleepiness, trouble concentrating, or behavioral and mood changes.

2. *Parasomnias—sleepwalking, sleep talking, and night terrors*

What are they?

A parasomnia is an unpleasant or undesirable event that intrudes into sleep but that doesn't change the quality or quantity of sleep a person gets. The most common parasomnias that we see in kids are sleepwalking, sleep talking, confusional arousals, and night terrors.

What causes them?

We categorize parasomnias according to what phase of sleep they happen in. Serious parasomnias that happen in REM sleep are rare, but this is the part of sleep that nightmares come from, so technically you will deal with a REM parasomnia many times in your life. More common are non-REM (NREM) parasomnias, which occur during a phase of sleep called "N3," a part of sleep that we have the most of during the first third of sleep (which explains why most kids start sleepwalking, sleep talking, or have night terrors earlier in the night.)

The exact cause of NREM parasomnias isn't known, but scientists have some ideas why they occur. It's thought that because the boundaries between sleep and wake are still maturing in kids, they're more susceptible to these conditions. There's some evidence that these issues are genetic, too. NREM parasomnias happen more when sleep is fragmented, which you can see in children who have sleep apnea, are in pain, or otherwise experience lower quality sleep. They can also happen without any obvious trigger.

How common are they?

NREM parasomnias are the most common sleep disorder in children. Around 30 percent of kids will have at least one episode of sleepwalking, and as many as 50 percent of parents report an episode or more of sleep talking in their children. Night terrors and confusional arousals are also common, affecting approximately 7 and 17 percent of children, respectively. Most NREM parasomnias go away on their own, typically by a kid's twelfth birthday.

What are the symptoms?

Most kids are completely unaware of these events. It's something that parents and family members notice, and the symptoms are different depending on the diagnosis. Sleepwalkers walk, sleep talkers talk. Night terrors and confusional arousals are characterized by periods of waking up, usually sitting up in bed, and seeming distressed. Kids can cry, moan, whimper, say words like "no" or "go away," and are inconsolable. Eyes tend to stay closed, and there aren't major physical symptoms other than facial flushing, sweating, or agitation. The episodes can last anywhere from a few minutes to a half hour (or occasionally more). When the event is over, kids go right back to sleep as if nothing happened.

3. Allergies, asthma, and viral illnesses

What are they?

One of the most common reasons kids have medical sleep disturbances actually isn't from a primary sleep disorder.

Rather, a large number of kids who have problems sleeping that aren't due to a typical sleep regression end up being diagnosed with allergies, asthma, or a viral illness.

What causes them?
Any cold virus can interrupt sleep, and the cough that lingers for weeks after the initial illness can continue to cause issues. Asthma and environmental allergies can have nighttime symptoms, with congestion, coughing, and trouble breathing all making it hard to get a good night's sleep.

How common are they?
Viruses are universal. During the toddler years, it's possible to have a new cold virus every few weeks (which translates to near continuous sniffles for the entire viral season). Not all viruses cause sleep problems, and your pediatrician will be able to sort out, over time, if a cold is the best explanation for the symptoms you notice. Asthma is a common pediatric diagnosis, estimated to affect around 6 percent of children in the United States. Environmental allergies are even more common in kids, with as many as one in five children in the United States carrying this diagnosis.

What are the symptoms?
Any overnight breathing issues, chest tightness, coughing, sneezing, snoring can be part of a bigger picture of asthma, allergies, or viral infection. Your pediatrician will piece it all together to see what diagnosis makes the most sense, and if there's any testing or treatment you should pursue.

Transitioning Out of a Crib—When, Why, and How

One of the most common sleep-related questions I get during the toddler years is a simple one: When should I transition my child from a crib to a bed? The simple answer—that there's no right answer—can feel frustrating but should also be liberating. There's no deadline for a transition out of a crib, and as with everything, only you will know when this change makes sense for your child (and for you!).

There are some developmental and logistical considerations that can guide you. At some point, your kid will be tall enough to break free—often catapulting themselves over the crib railing and leading to some stressful, usually minor injuries. This is one of the few obvious indications that it's time to get that toddler bed ready, take down that removable crib wall, or set up whatever unenclosed sleep space you plan on making. A regular bed with a rail and some mats to cushion falls (and help getting into and out of bed), a toddler bed, or a floor pillow setup are all equally fine choices.

Barring safety concerns, you'll make your decision based on your own unique risk-and-benefit assessment. Some kids aren't in any rush to get out of their crib. I consider myself to be in this lucky camp, with a toddler daughter who woke up at 6:00 a.m. but happily sang and played in her crib for another hour or more while her parents caught a few more Z's. Other crib sleepers scream bloody murder until you retrieve them, but once you take down the removable crib wall they decide to play in their room patiently and give you some additional, magical morning rest. Still, others will wake you in the early morning no matter what—either crying for you to get them from their crib or running into your bed to cajole you out.

Your own sleep needs, your child's temperament, their developmental level, and their own motivation (some toddlers proactively ask for big-kid beds, especially if they see an older sibling with one!) will determine when you make the change. As a final consideration, don't forget to factor your toilet training journey into the equation. As we discussed, lots of kids stay in overnight Pull-Ups for months or years after they are successfully toilet trained. But even if you still find wet Pull-Ups in the morning, there's a good chance your kid is physically able to stay dry overnight. Kids who wake up in cribs will rarely wait for you to put them on the toilet for that first morning pee. Even in a bed, kids often wake up and use their Pull-Up out of convenience rather than journey to the toilet on their own. Transitioning to a bed doesn't guarantee overnight continence, and keeping your toilet trained toddler in their crib with Pull-Ups is a very reasonable choice. When you decide to work on staying dry overnight, however, make sure it's after you've made the crib-to-bed transition.

THE BOTTOM LINE

5 out of 5 Pediatrician Parents Agree

1. Toddler sleep issues are extremely common. The most frequently encountered sleep regressions involve overnight awakenings and bedtime struggles. These are often set off by illnesses or life changes but can happen without any identifiable trigger.

2. Many, many sleep regressions go away on their own. It's okay to wait it out and see how things settle (especially if your little one is sick or stressed) before you dive into troubleshooting mode.

3. Sleep is all connected. The best strategies to improve overnight awakenings frequently involve refocusing efforts on bedtime routines. Every child is different, and only you will know which aspects of your child's sleep schedule could use improvement and which techniques make sense to try.

4. A bedtime pass (a ticket your toddler relinquishes to gain entry into your bed but earns them a prize if they don't use it) is a nice way to start motivating your toddler to sleep on their own overnight—if and when that's something you want to try!

5. There are lots of medical reasons your child may be having issues with getting the sleep they need. If you feel this might be the case—or aren't sure—talk to your pediatrician. The most common conditions that we diagnose and treat are parasomnias (like sleepwalking, sleep talking, night terrors), asthma, allergies, and obstructive sleep apnea.

6. Only you will know the best time to transition your toddler from a crib to a bed. Physical safety (e.g., toddlers who catapult themselves out of their crib in escape attempts) and overnight toilet training may signal that it's time to make the change. Otherwise, you'll transition when you and your little one are both ready!

PART THREE

HEALTH + SOCIETY

CHAPTER 10

THE DOC IS IN

Who Ya Gonna Call?
(Your Pediatrician!)

I have a confession: I get nervous before doctor's visits. I know, I'm a doctor! And a pediatrician (hence the subtitle of this book). So it's even wilder to admit that I get just as nervous for my daughter's appointments.

As I tell my daughter, I really do understand that the pediatrician is our friend, and I'm eager to get my kid medical care and attention. But mom anxiety trumps reason, and I often find myself worrying about what the visit will entail, if anything will be "wrong," or if I'll feel bad about any of my parenting choices.

Don't get me wrong—I know my pediatrician isn't there to judge. I also know my daughter will be just fine with the poking and prodding. There isn't a ton of logic to the anxiety (when is there ever?). It's just one of my things, and maybe it's one of yours, too. Or maybe it's not, but you're looking for some ways to make doctor's visits a little less stressful for your little one. Either way, I'm here to help prepare everyone. Knowing what to expect is (at least!) half the battle.

This chapter is a crash course in pediatrician visits. Yes, you've been to more than your fair share during your baby's first year, but now things are different. Hopefully you've been empowered to say yes to every life-saving childhood vaccine according to the recommended life-saving schedule. Watching your baby cry was tough, and those early fevers and fusses were no picnic, either. But now, your kid is smarter, older, bigger, and with a much better memory. They will likely have some deep feelings about what a doctor's visit entails, and preparing them will take more than bringing a post-shot bottle or breast and stocking up on infant Tylenol.

And as routine checkups become much less frequent— spacing out to as little as once a year!—it's even more important to remind yourself that you can call your pediatrician anytime. Not just for crises (if you haven't already followed your instinct and brought your little one to the emergency room if needed), but for the everyday bumps in the road that will almost certainly fall your way. I'll break down the most common reasons you'll make a special visit to your kid's doctor, and some expert tips that can guide your discussion.

Time for Your Checkup

Here are some tips for preparing your little one—and the whole family—for the lowest-stress checkups possible.

1. Prepare yourself first.

You may have noticed that, among the many themes of this book, the idea of looking at your own feelings and reactions first is a big one. While I knew this would be important work when it came to the big behavioral topics like separation anxiety and tantrums, it was less instinctive to apply it elsewhere. But it's important nonetheless and makes things easier as you go forward into the next steps.

This might just mean taking a minute to acknowledge that watching your little one cry when they get their vaccines understandably upsets you. Maybe it's a deeper, messier anxiety about physician visits that you have to untangle. No matter what the stress may be, let yourself be a parent and have your own feelings. It will help you feel psychologically prepared and will do wonders in modeling emotional awareness and resilience to your child.

Some logistical preparation is helpful, too. You should feel empowered to make sooner appointments for specific concerns. But chances are that you'll still have some questions for the pediatrician when it's time for the well-child visit, so write them down and bring them with you.

2. Prepare together.

In our first chapters, we talked a lot about setting a solid foundation when it comes to behavioral struggles. You've spent time and energy in thoughtfully modeling emotional regulation, teaching coping strategies when frustrations arise, and building your child's resilience arsenal. It's work that will translate into specific stressors like doctor's visits. Review the techniques from those chapters and remember that you are more prepared than you think.

In addition to general emotional regulation, you can start to work specifically on addressing your kid's doctor anxiety. This doesn't have to be a chore, and it really shouldn't be! Think of it instead as an opportunity and focus on the positive parts of preparation. Specifically, it's helpful to read books, watch shows, and play games that familiarize your child with the process of seeing the doctor. *Doc McStuffins* was a godsend, doing a ton of heavy lifting in the background (yes, we sang "Time for Your Checkup" before examining stuffed animals and even on the way to my daughter's own well-child visits). High-quality media and books that normalize doctor's visits are abundant and incredibly useful.

Playtime gives you a great opportunity to add your two cents, too. No need to be heavy-handed and excessively editorialize, but feel free to add in some commentary. We talked all the time about how important it was to see the doctor, which of course came up more in our household than most as my daughter started to ask questions about what Mommy does at work. Even if your child isn't related to anyone who "fixes babies," there will be plenty of chances to normalize checkups. You'll quickly notice that doctor-themed pretend play takes off on its own; stuffed animals will get shots and dolls will need medicine. Lean into it and have fun. That's your top priority. If the opportunity to more overtly insert scripted preparation arises—"It's normal to be nervous at the doctor, Teddy Bear, but you're safe and it's important to get a checkup to stay healthy. Mommy's here if you need a hug"—I'm sure you'll take it.

3. Pack your supplies.

As with so many things in life, the hardest part of going to the doctor is frequently the anticipation. I let my daughter know we were going for a checkup the night before, then reminded her the next morning. Then I packed the supplies we would need to make the in-office waiting process as painless as possible. Tablets, toys, books, snacks—bring whatever you need to make the waiting game easier.

I also found that letting my daughter bring a stuffed animal or doll to get a checkup with her was extremely helpful. A special doll and a toy doctor kit (stethoscope, otoscope, and all) came with us to every visit. Pediatricians will happily accommodate this—and almost anything—that facilitates enough cooperation to perform a good physical exam.

I also was pretty indulgent in my post-visit prizes. The doctor usually had stickers, but I brought a backup just in case. I was (and still am) a big fan of giving books as presents, so a $5 board book was the perfect reward, and something that came with us to the visit. She knew she would get stickers and a prize after her shots, and quickly started telling her stuffed animals that they would get imaginary versions of these rewards after each pretend checkup was complete.

4. Tell the truth. Always.

It's tempting to hide the truth when you know your kid is about to deal with something painful, no matter how temporary. The instinct is common, but it's counterproductive. We know from work with hospitalized children that lying about stressors to come causes more harm than good. There's no need for a prolonged speech, just a simple warning shot (pun intended). I told my daughter during all our preparation and pretend play that shots "hurt for a moment, and it's okay to cry. I'll keep hugging you and you'll be safe. It's okay to cry as much as you want. We have to do this so you can stay healthy. Afterward we can get a sticker and a book prize."

5. Claim bragging rights.

When it's done, celebrate! Your kid—and you—did a great job. No matter how much they cried, they still got the evaluation and preventive care they need to be healthy. It's a big win, so shout it out loud. We went through our contact list as soon as we got home, FaceTiming friends, grandparents, cousins, anyone who was ready to hear how we absolutely nailed our checkup.

Acute Issues, Urgent Visits, and When You'll Be Calling Your Pediatrician

I've said it once (or many more times) and I'll say it again: You can call your pediatrician with any concern. As well-child visits become less frequent, it's even more likely that you'll have items to discuss in between visits. In general, it's better for everyone to schedule a special appointment just to tackle those topics. It helps you get answers more quickly, and it helps you and your pediatrician have more dedicated time to address specific issues. Questions about sleep, eating, behavior—any nonurgent issue we discussed in the previous chapters merits its own visit. Your concern is reason enough to make an appointment.

When it comes to urgent issues, I have a simple rule: If you're wondering whether to call the pediatrician, just call the pediatrician. There is no need to waste time and energy looking at Google, texting friends, or asking your local Facebook group if a medical concern needs medical evaluation. If you're worried enough to wonder what's going on, go straight to the doctor. It may not need same-day evaluation, but it's not your job to decide that. Let the medical professionals make medical decisions, and focus on just being a parent.

And if you think it's an emergency that can't wait for the on-call callback (or aren't sure), then it's an emergency! You'll go to the ER, call 911, or otherwise get the immediate help you need. I've seen countless patients in the emergency room whose parents apologized when the issue turned out to be, technically, in hindsight, not emergent. My answer was always the same: Please don't apologize! My job is to promote pediatric health. Safe children who aren't critically ill make me happy, not angry. Providing a basic workup and reassurance is just as much a part of my job as treating severely sick kids.

It takes years of medical school, then pediatric residency, to get even a basic list of the reasons you may be calling your pediatrician. I couldn't go through them all here even if I wanted to! Instead, let's cover some of the most common semi-urgent, urgent, and emergent issues that pediatricians treat. As a bonus, I'll add in some strategies you can try while waiting for that on-call provider to get back to you.

1. Colds, cough, viral illnesses, diarrhea, and fevers

Happy first birthday, little one! The world has decided to generously gift your toddler a never-ending onslaught of viral illnesses. As in, a new cold every few weeks and a new normal where constant sneezing, sniffles, cough, and congestion is the rule, not the exception.

This is one of the most challenging triage topics I see parents deal with: When is a cold bad enough to see the doctor? When do I need to bring my kid to the emergency room? And of course, is there anything I can do at home to help them?

The simplest, safest, and overall best answer to the first two questions is: You'll call your pediatrician when you're worried. You'll run to the emergency room when it's an emergency. Each medical situation is different, and there isn't any strict one-size-fits-all playbook I can give here that will safely triage every possible situation. Calling your pediatrician when you're unsure, and calling 911 when your emergency spidey sense is tingling, is the way to go.

That said, there are a few signs to be aware of. Red flags indicating that a trip to the emergency room is the likely answer are when your congested kid starts breathing really fast, when their skin starts to suck in between their ribs or into their neck, when their nostrils start flaring, or when it's otherwise clear they are having trouble breathing. If it's not an emergency, you'll be able to comfort your child at home—even if it's just while waiting for your pediatrician to let you know if and when you need to bring them in. After the age of twelve months honey is safe to give, and scientifically proven to suppress coughs. It works better than cough medicine, and we don't give over-the-counter cold medicine to young kids anyway—they have lots of side effects that make any potential benefit unlikely to be worthwhile. Bulb suctioning can be helpful for congestion that's bothering your little one, and some people love slightly more intense devices like the NoseFrida. Over-the-counter saline drops in the nose help some babies, too, and steam is almost always useful. While lots of families like nebulizer machines with humidified salt water (which is a fine option), I favor a simpler approach. I recommend parents run a hot shower in a closed bathroom, let the room fill with steam, then bring their little one in for a brief steam room session.

Other tried-and-true cold remedies include plenty of snuggles, lots of rest (screen time is unlimited during every illness in my house), and acetaminophen (Tylenol) or ibuprofen (Motrin) for discomfort and fevers. Popsicles are great for throat pain, and can also help keep kids hydrated. Another common reason kids are brought in for medical care when they have a cold is dehydration. We think of this with stomach viruses—which you'll likely deal with as well—but even an upper-respiratory virus can cause enough malaise and stomach discomfort (or make it hard enough to breathe and eat at the same time) that hydration becomes an issue. Diarrhea happens with any type of virus, making dehydration even more likely. Keeping track of wet diapers is helpful. A good benchmark to remember is that not having a wet diaper for eight hours usually warrants a call to your kid's doctor. You'll do your best to offer fluids in whatever form your little one will take, and bring them in if they just can't keep up.

2. Rashes, injuries, and new body findings

It's easy to forget where the word "toddler" comes from. It's as intuitive as it seems: toddlers toddle. As they learn to walk, they wobble and fall down. Even when they've gained some steadiness, coordination is still developing. Lumps, bumps, bruises, scrapes, and all sorts of injuries are something that all toddler parents deal with at some point. If you're concerned about a broken bone, or have a head injury that needs to be checked for a concussion, bring your little one right to the emergency room and let the doctors take it from there.

Just as common as toddler injuries are toddler skin changes. You're likely to find new rashes, marks, and assorted dermatologic findings on more occasions than you can count. With the exception of the hives that come with anaphylaxis (a severe allergic reaction) and a few very rare skin disorders, rashes tend not to be an emergency. But even if there's no emergent concern, there's still no reason to turn to Google or sit in worry until your next well-child visit. Call your pediatrician and see if they want to see your kid today, tomorrow, or in the next few weeks. While you wait for your visit, take pictures and note any other symptoms. Keep an eye out for any possible triggers. If things change, or new concerning findings pop up, know you can always seek evaluation sooner.

3. *Constipation*

It may seem unbalanced to give constipation its own special shoutout after lumping all sorts of other illnesses and body changes together, but constipation is such a common, frustrating issue for toddlers that it's only fair to pay it a little extra attention.

In *Parent like a Pediatrician*, we talked about baby constipation in a lot of detail. Many of the same principles apply to toddlers—especially when it comes to frequency. The internet may try to convince you that your child's weekly bowel movement signals constipation, but it's not that simple. It doesn't really matter how often your little one poops, and some kids are perfectly happy and healthy going every eight days (really!). It's when bowel movements are hard, even pellet-like, that constipation is the clear diagnosis. Also, unlike babies, not-constipated toddlers don't tend to strain, grunt, or turn red, adding these signs to the list of reasons you should call your pediatrician.

The potential causes of constipation are vast, and it's frequently multifactorial. The most common triggers for toddler constipation are suboptimal hydration, inadequate dietary fiber, and the process of toileting itself. If you're troubleshooting at home, your pediatrician will likely have you focus on offering your kid more fluids to drink, offering higher fiber foods, and making a few adjustments to toilet time. As kids learn to control their bowels, it's hard for them to find the balance between holding until they can go to the bathroom and holding on too long. Many toddlers have anxiety about toileting, especially bowel movements, which worsens this withholding behavior. Scheduling times to sit on the toilet—with feet on the ground—can be a very helpful strategy. (If you feel like you've been set up with a series of conflicting, impossible tasks, I hear you. Don't push your kid to sit on the toilet or potty train, but also have timed toilet sits for their constipation. Don't force food or drink and trust them to get the hydration and nutrition they deserve, but also make sure they have enough fluids and fiber. It's a variation of our favorite theme: that there's no right or wrong, safe or unsafe, and instead that everything is a balance of risk and benefit.)

There are plenty of times when none of this works, or your child won't cooperate. In these cases, there's a very good chance that your pediatrician will recommend a laxative (MiraLAX is extremely safe and effective at this age) or a fiber supplement. It's not a sign of failure, and you'll do what you need to do to get through your individual situation.

THE BOTTOM LINE

5 out of 5 Pediatrician Parents Agree

1. Anxiety about pediatrician visits is normal—both for toddlers and their parents! Validate your own worry and remember all the groundwork you've set for emotional regulation already.

2. On-topic books, shows, and working through doctor anxiety in your pretend play can do wonders in getting your toddler ready for their checkup. Pack your supplies—books, toys, dolls (whom your pediatrician will happily examine alongside your child), snacks, post-shot prizes—the night before, and remind your child that the next day's routine includes a doctor's visit.

3. Tell the truth, always, especially when it comes to poking and prodding. It's tempting to say shots won't hurt, but this is a lie. Remind your child it's okay to be scared, it's okay to cry, and that you'll be there for hugs and prizes. And make sure you both brag far and wide, to family and friends, about the day's bravery after you're done!

4. You can call your pediatrician about anything, always. As check-ups become less frequent, visits to discuss specific issues become even more important. And when it comes to emergencies, you can keep it simple: don't pass Go, don't collect $200, do *not* go to your local Facebook group. Just call 911, or bring your child to the emergency room, if you feel they may need immediate medical evaluation.

5. Common "chief complaints" that bring toddlers into the pediatrician office are coughs, colds, rashes, injuries, and constipation. If these present in the form of an emergency—such as viruses that cause labored breathing, allergic reactions, and bone/head injuries—you'll be going to the emergency room instead!

6. If you're in the nonemergency zone, fight the urge to crowdsource solutions on social media and instead call your pediatrician. While you wait for a callback from the on-call doc or scheduler, you can try humidified air for colds, honey for coughs, and collect data (including photos!) about rashes.

7. Constipation is super common in the toddler years, and there's a good chance you'll embrace dietary fiber, timed toileting, hydration, and even MiraLAX at some point.

CHAPTER 11

NATURAL DISASTER

Your Toddler Still Doesn't Need Kombucha (or Any Unregulated Remedies or Supplements, but They Sure Do Need Their Vaccines!)

In an age of increasing distrust with our for-profit medical system, parents express understandable anxiety that there are just too many medications, tests, pokes, and shots these days. It's true. We have more treatments than ever, and people—kids included—visit doctors more frequently. It's a complex issue, and there are times when I agree little kids are given medical treatments that they either don't really need, or can even be harmful!

But I'm still a pediatrician, and remain a believer in modern medicine, which has done wonders to help children lead long and healthy lives. There's room for a balanced discussion, understanding that "traditional" medicine has an

important role even for the tiniest patients, while acknowledging that overtreating is definitely a real issue. However,
the booming "alternative" market (let's call them Big Nature
to match their Big Pharma counterparts) has forced a far less
nuanced conversation: ditch "traditional" medicine altogether and go the route of the "natural." There continue to
be an obscene number of unregulated and risky treatments
targeted specifically to anxious parents. Most of them are, at
best, unproven, and, at worst, plain dangerous.

Where does that leave you, my savvy, caring parent?
It's time to revisit my framework on approaching "natural"
remedies. This comes with a refresher on the pesky little
naturalistic fallacy (nope, natural is *not* always better) that
keeps getting in the way of safe, scientific, and commonsense
parenting choices. Debunking the naturalistic fallacy will
give us the perfect opportunity to bust anti-vaccine propaganda, a movement that is deeply steeped in oversimplified
"pro-natural" movements, and with catastrophic results.

Let's start by reviewing the approach I use when counseling parents on whether a nontraditional treatment makes
sense. If you use these guiding questions in your discussion
with your own pediatrician, and for self-reflection, you'll be
able to make the smartest, safest choices for your child.

1. Remember that "natural" is a myth.

"Natural" does not mean safer, and at an atomic level, there's
no meaningful difference between "natural" and "chemical"

products. You see, the thing about molecules is that it doesn't really matter where they came from. The human body handles the active ingredient from a tea, plant, oil, or tincture exactly the same as it handles a synthesized compound designed to mimic the plant it was discovered in (which accounts for the majority of all pharmaceutical treatments). It may be easy to trick our minds, but our bodies see everything that we put into them as medicine. And all medicines have risks and benefits. It's also key to remember that "natural," however arbitrary the definition may be, does *not* mean "better." Babies used to die all the time before modern medicine from "natural" things like dysentery and even common colds. They still do.

2. Does my kid need treatment at all?

When approaching any alternative remedy, the first step is to ask yourself: Is something actually wrong? Does my kid need to take medicine?

Remember that everything that your child ingests is a medicine and comes with risk, no matter how small. It's not possible to say that something is necessary, effective, important without also acknowledging that this makes it, by definition, a medical treatment with real risks and benefits. For now, there's no evidence that any available supplement actually helps children when given routinely. So while it's easy to take a "Why not?" approach to these seemingly low-risk supplements and give them just in case, science (and common sense) really don't support this. Starting the discussion with the first, fundamental question of whether your kid actually needs treatment has been a complete game changer for me, and for so many parents.

3. Who is saying my kid needs this treatment?

Hear about it from a friend? Did they see it on their social media feed? Maybe it wasn't an actual #ad, but there was a link that gave the promoter a commission, or maybe there's a partnership they didn't even disclose. In a world full of health influencers, it's harder than ever to fully understand the motivation behind any parenting recommendation. Sorting through supplements, treatments, and "holistic" options for your little one has become almost impossible. Is this genuine advice? Unscrupulous, predatory advertising? Something in between? It's challenging for even the savviest scroller to know for sure.

And despite how much a promoter may genuinely believe in any product, it's impossible to be completely objective when financial gains are at stake. Online, I refuse to promote products for profit (even ones I genuinely adore) because I know that it will cloud my objectivity. It's why in medicine, our days are filled with financial disclosure forms, investigations into conflicts of interest, and constant introspection into how we can provide the best, most honest information possible without succumbing to undue influence. So, keep your expectations high for the integrity of traditional medicine and healthcare corporations, and raise them just as high for anyone promoting a "natural" product.

4. Has this treatment been tested? How and by whom?

The simple truth is that any "alternative" remedy just won't come with a lot of good science behind it. Some of that is Big Nature evading rigorous evaluation to maximize profit, but some of it is also traditional medicine's fault. We've been reluctant to study alternative products for a variety of reasons (Big Pharma, racism, xenophobia, arrogance, funding), and it's something we're trying to fix. There are more and more studies to determine if these treatments are safe and effective, and we have better evidence to guide our recommendations each day. The reality, though, is that this data is still sparse, and even when we do have studies, it's much harder to draw conclusions about safety and efficacy. The world of "natural" products still lags when it comes to transparency, and there's a ton of variety in how remedies are made and used. So, while we don't always know exactly which ingredients are in a particular product or which methods are being used in a particular treatment, they may go by the exact same name. This lack of consistency makes it extremely hard to design a study that accurately compares equivalent "traditional" treatments. As a result, the studies we do have available, of which there are very few (*especially* for younger children), are much lower quality than we would hope for, and that much harder to draw conclusions from.

For supplements and "natural" remedies, a lack of appropriate regulation also makes safety a real concern. The majority of these products have, through very clever lobbying, been able to classify themselves as "dietary supplements" and escape the rigorous FDA review that "pharmaceuticals" must go through. This means that these products go through exactly zero external review of safety beyond their own, conflict-of-interest filled testing. I can't imagine anyone (myself included!) feeling comfortable with traditional pharmaceutical company's safety approval process consisting of self-reporting their own data to the FDA. And there is absolutely as much potential for improper regulation leading to real harm when it comes to so-called dietary supplements.

The lack of data and regulation means that it will always be more challenging to decide if an "alternative" treatment is the right choice. It's why I remind myself, my friends, and the families I counsel to spend extra time reflecting on whether any treatment is really needed at all. If it is, I lay out all possible remedies together, "traditional" and "alternative" alike. Once I've gathered as much information as possible about each, I'm better able to weigh my options side by side. Again, just like all pharmaceuticals, "natural" remedies have risks and benefits that need to be assessed—and compared to "traditional" medications that, simply by being better studied and more tightly regulated, are frequently better, safer options. Talk to your pediatrician and work through this together. Even if they ultimately recommend the pharmaceutical option, a savvy pediatrician will be able to help you assess what limited data we have on "alternatives" and help you make your own personal, big-picture risk versus benefit decision. And if you do decide that an unregulated product is something you want to explore, make sure to be even more cautious, even more skeptical, and even more critical of the safety and efficacy claims you see.

Rapid-Fire Vaccine Review

Let me just say it very clearly: Childhood vaccines are still safe and not to be missed—including flu and covid shots!

There's no greater victim of the naturalistic fallacy than health-affirming, life-saving childhood vaccines. Anti-vaccine misinformation isn't a monolith; there are plenty of motivations behind vaccine hesitancy, and it's not as simple as saying all vaccine opponents are pure science deniers. But the majority of anti-vaccine propaganda does originate from select Big Nature sources, who use the naturalistic fallacy to sell supplements and subscriptions. And regardless of the technique or intention, the reason that vaccine misinformation is so effective is the naturalistic fallacy. Our brains are hardwired to worry about "unnatural" products and trust "natural" alternatives.

As true as all of this is, knowing that Big Nature is taking advantage of our natural tendency is not enough to override the suspicion and distrust. We simply *will* ourselves out of an adaptive evolutionary psychological process, even when it's being exploited for harm. So let's review some of those anti-vaccine lies. In my first book, we took a deep, glorious dive into vaccine science and hopefully it helped you feel empowered to just say yes to vaccines without unnecessary stress. But if you still have questions, are new to my take on this topic, or fresh concerns have come up, that's more than okay! Let's briefly recap why anti-vaccine propaganda just doesn't hold up, and make your immunization angst a thing of the past.

1. Vaccines don't cause autism.

If you're still fretting over any possible links to autism, made famous by the measles-mumps-rubella (MMR) vaccine and the now thoroughly disgraced and debunked claims of Andrew Wakefield, one of medicine's greatest frauds, this is an easy one. Wakefield had multiple conflicts of interest, including financial gain from a competing vaccine maker, and created a falsified report to make it look like the MMR vaccine du jour was linked to autism. To put things in perspective, Wakefield's paper was a series of case reports (not even a study or trial) stating that twelve children who received the MMR vaccine later were diagnosed with autism. Let's compare that to a more recent analysis in 2014 that included data from more than one million (yes, a million) children and found exactly zero relationship.

2. *Alternative schedules are a hard pass.*

Why are there so many more new vaccines than there were when you were a kid? And couldn't all these shots hurt a baby and overwhelm their tiny immune system? The simple answer is that there are more vaccines because science is awesome and we've been able to invent amazing life-saving immunizations at a fairly rapid rate. What's more, even though we now have vaccines for more diseases, we've been able to engineer them better, using fewer antigens, which is the part of the vaccine that mimics a virus or bacterium and triggers an immune response. I tell parents, accurately, that one visit for vaccines exposes their kid to fewer antigens than if their toddler touched a doorknob and then licked their hand. (And they will do this and touch far grimier things very frequently and from a very young age.) And all vaccines have fewer antigens than the actual diseases, so it is much more "overwhelming" for a baby's immune system to see a real-life virus or bacterium than to be vaccinated.

Okay, but isn't it stressful for kids to have so many shots all at once? Many parents wonder about "alternative schedules," and feel that giving fewer vaccines at each visit is less traumatic for their little ones. But science disagrees. New studies show that giving all the vaccines at once is actually less stressful for a child because it's fewer separate instances of giving shots. And children who receive several vaccines at the same time don't have any more side effects or complications compared to children who get only one shot at a time. More important, the current CDC schedule has been designed based on decades of research to create the safest and most protective vaccination plan for children. Babies have the weakest immune systems during their first year of life, as they begin to lose protection from their mother's antibodies that cross through the placenta. So we vaccinate as soon as it's safe and effective to do so, protecting babies during a time when they are the most vulnerable.

3. Vaccine ingredients are safe.

I promise you that each component in every childhood vaccine is both necessary and completely safe. Predatory anti-vaccine groups have been devious in their ability to co-opt anxiety about the unknown, and the list of ingredients in vaccines have complex and frankly scary-sounding names that can terrify even the savviest parent. Anti-vax websites instruct parents to ask their pediatrician to review each item on the vaccine insert, promising a "gotcha" moment proving how dangerous they really are. But I review these ingredients in my daily practice when I counsel families, and I've never been "got."

For a comprehensive review of vaccine ingredients, check out *Parent Like a Pediatrician*, or click through the links on my website (the Children's Hospital of Philadelphia vaccine education center has a phenomenal guide). Here's a quick recap to remind you why vaccine ingredients are safe and important—yes, all of them.

VACCINE INGREDIENTS 101

Antigens

Examples: See "A Is for Antigen" later in this chapter.

How they work/what they do: Each vaccine contains an active ingredient, known as an "antigen," which is the part of the vaccine that allows the body to create an immune response. This part of the vaccine is either a whole virus or bacterium, a portion of a virus or bacterium, a chemical that the bacteria makes when it infects a person, or (excitingly and recently!) a genetic building block that tells your body to make an immune-generating viral protein.

Why they're safe: The main concern I hear from parents about "antigens" is whether they can cause an actual infection. It's a good question, since they can contain actual parts of a bacterium or virus that causes serious illness. The short answer is no, the longer answer is in the "antigen" chart.

Adjuvant

Examples: In the United States, the three adjuvants used in vaccines are aluminum salts, monophosphoryl lipid A, and squalene.

How they work/what they do: Adjuvants are substances that make the vaccine work better by causing a stronger immune response. This means that fewer doses of a vaccine are needed, and/or that we can give a smaller dose of the vaccine to your baby.

Why they're safe: Some anti-vaccine groups focus on aluminum, claiming that because it's a metal that makes it "toxic" and dangerous. Nope. The fun fact they ignore is that humans consume metals *all the time*. Those healthy "vitamins and minerals" that your breakfast cereal contains? Those minerals are zinc, copper, iron, selenium, manganese, and other trace metals. Aluminum isn't a metal that your body needs in the same way, but it is absolutely found in normal foods and something we consume every day. Another fun fact: in the first six months of life, infants get more aluminum from breastmilk or formula than they do from receiving all the routine vaccines combined.

Stabilizers

Examples: Gelatin, polysorbate 80

How they work/what they do: These are substances (sometimes just run-of-the-mill food products like gelatin) that help vaccines last during production and transport.

Why they're safe: We think that stabilizers might be the component of vaccines that are responsible for extremely rare (as in more than one in one million chance) serious but treatable allergic reactions. They don't have any other side effects. Of course, that doesn't mean they haven't been the target of misinformation. When the amazing, cancer-preventing HPV vaccine came out, claims quickly emerged that its stabilizer, polysorbate 80, causes infertility. It doesn't. Polysorbate 80 is another crossover from the food industry and has been used in ice cream production for many years. A typical serving of ice cream has about 170,000 micrograms of polysorbate 80. Each dose of the HPV vaccine contains 50 micrograms.

Preservatives

Examples: Thimerosal

How they work/what they do: This type of ingredient is something you find in multidose vials, and this makes sense. Since we want these multiple-use containers to last longer, we need to add preservatives. Preservatives are extremely important and prevent contamination from other bacteria or even fungi. This was a big problem with the early vaccines, but thankfully contaminated vaccines are a worry of the past.

Why they're safe: The most famous preservative, thimerosal, became a topic of great controversy when Wakefield's acolytes proposed it was the ingredient linked to autism. Extensive research has proved this to be false, but even so, in 1999 the FDA recommended removing thimerosal from all childhood vaccines in the United States (with the exception of the multidose vial of the influenza vaccine) "just in case," in an attempt to end the vaccine "debate" once and for all. By caving to anti-vaccine lobbies, scientists believed they could close the conversation. Instead, the anti-vaccine propaganda machine used this decision as ammunition to claim a victory, stating that thimerosal had been dangerous all along. And almost immediately, these anti-vaccine groups found new vaccine components to make erroneous and fear-based claims about. Trust the science: you don't have to worry about thimerosal or the multidose flu shot.

A Is for Antigen

There are five main ways that scientists can make an antigen that lets the body learn how to fight a disease without ever seeing an actual living organism.

1. *Subunit, conjugate, polysaccharide, or recombinant.* These are all words that describe the same concept: Scientists take just one component of the bacterium or virus—the part that the human body recognizes when it gets an infection and uses to make immune cells and memory—and isolate it from the rest of the virus or bacterium's disease-causing badness. There's no way your kid can get sick from these vaccines—like, ever—because there's no part of the vaccine that knows how to reproduce and infect their body.

2. *Toxoid.* These work in pretty much the exact same way as antigens that come from just part of a virus or bacterium, but instead of using part of the organism they use the "toxin" it makes. Don't get scared by this word! It's not anything that's toxic to your baby's body. Some very horrible diseases—famously tetanus and diphtheria, truly horrific illnesses that I thankfully have never seen—make a toxin when they infect you, and this is what your immune system fights when it gets sick. Again, there isn't any part of the bacterium or virus in these vaccines that can reproduce and get into your cells, so it's not possible to actually get tetanus or diphtheria from it. It's literally never happened.

3. *Inactivated.* The third method of making sure an antigen isn't active at all is . . . to inactivate it. This really just means killing the bacterium or virus so that all the immune-producing parts are there, but it loses all its powers to infect you. How do we know this process works? Sadly, it's from an extremely and famously horrible historical incident when this process went wrong. In 1955, hundreds of thousands of the brand-new, life-saving polio vaccines managed to leave the factory after a defective inactivation process. About forty thousand children contracted polio from the vaccine, two hundred were seriously ill, and ten died. It's an incredible tragedy that happened very, very early in our nation's vaccine-manufacturing process. It's one of the many reasons the FDA is so strict about vaccine oversight, and there have been exactly zero cases of faulty inactivation since then.

4. *Live-attenuated.* Some vaccines do still contain very small amounts of technically "alive" virus in them. These are called "live-attenuated," and the only routine childhood vaccines that fall into this category are the MMR vaccine (measles, mumps, and rubella), varicella (chicken pox), and rotavirus. The best part of these vaccines is that the immunity your baby gets from them lasts a lot longer, so the vast majority of kids won't need any boosters at all when they grow up. The only downside is that for someone with an extremely weak immune system, they can "reactivate" and cause actual disease.

Stressed? No need! The rotavirus vaccine is given orally to infants starting at two months. By then, any serious, extremely rare immune problem that makes this vaccine unsafe will be well-known to you and your doctor. In all of my years seeing sick kids in the hospital, I've seen only one case where this vaccine was skipped. It was a child with severe combined immune deficiency (SCID), an extremely uncommon but very serious disease that is picked up either on the newborn screen or in the first weeks of life. Otherwise, babies who get the rotavirus vaccine do great. And while rotavirus might sound like a no-big-deal viral stomach bug, it's actually no joke. When babies do have rotavirus, even with modern medicine and all the IV fluids I can give them, they are sick for days or weeks, requiring long hospital stays. And in other countries, viruses that cause diarrhea are actually the leading cause of death in infants. The MMR and varicella vaccines are similarly safe and are given for the first time at six to twelve months to be extra sure that babies have an immune system that is ready to handle them.

5. *mRNA and DNA.* The last, latest way to engineer an antigen is probably something you're already pretty familiar with. It's how those incredible new covid vaccines work. When the antigen is mRNA (like with the Moderna and Pfizer vaccines), this means delivering this protein-encoding piece of material to your body, where your cells will take it up and use it to create that now-famous spike protein themselves. The mRNA can't get into your DNA, into your RNA, or really

into anything. It's just a protein-making machine that lets your own human cells share the signal to create covid immunity—without ever having to see the actual big, bad covid-causing virus themselves!

The other way that scientists take advantage of viral genetic codes is what you see in the other covid vaccines, and it's a really similar concept. Instead of using mRNA to help your body prepare its immune system for a covid invasion, it uses DNA. The molecular properties of RNA and DNA are different. RNA is easily taken in by cells, but when DNA is the antigen, it needs a bit more help. So to aid cellular entry, scientists use something called a "viral vector." This actually doesn't have anything to do with the coronavirus itself. Instead, another common cold virus, most commonly "adenovirus," gets killed in a lab (RIP). Put some immunity-creating DNA in this deceased viral shell (which can't replicate or infect you but still knows how to enter cells) and you get the same result as any other antigen: your body sees something that belongs to the baddie you're trying to prevent and learns how to fight it.

4. It's never too late.

Really, it's okay to be late to the party. Did anti-vaccine propaganda catch you in your vulnerable postpartum state and you're late to the game? Maybe life just got in the way and somehow you missed a shot (or more)? Or perhaps you thought an alternative schedule made sense but now you see that a scientific schedule is the way to go? That's great! Your pediatrician should be *thrilled* to help your little one catch up. In fact, the CDC has a comprehensive "catch-up" schedule just for situations like this. Changing your mind when presented with new information is a sign of strength and growth. There shouldn't be any judgment—from yourself, your social circle, or your child's doctor—and you can still ask any and all questions about vaccines (or any other health topic!) that arise in the future.

5. Flu and covid vaccines are not to be missed.

If you've seen me preaching the wonders of seasonal virus vaccination out in the wild, you may wonder where my enthusiasm comes from—especially when the rollout for pediatric covid vaccines has been met with such a tepid response. Why am I so obsessed with the covid vaccines and why do I know that kids absolutely need to get their shots, just like adults? Because kids deserve protection from covid. Full stop. There's been way too much talk from pundits and politicians about if, how, and how much covid is a threat to kids. I understand wanting to keep worries in check. It's been a rough few years, to say the least. It's all too easy to get swept up in the endless anxiety. So a little perspective makes sense, and reminding yourself that your kid's exposure to covid isn't the be-all, end-all of possible dangers is important.

The truth is that parenting is full of dangers, difficult choices, risk-benefit balances. Every decision we make balances the potential harms with the potential gains. With covid, this means staying on task and weighing the risks of covid to kids with the risks of the measures we take to prevent it.

What are the risks of covid transmission and infection? They don't need to be panic inducing, but they're significant. Covid can affect children, and while the percentage of kids who get seriously sick from acute illness is much lower than adults, it's not zero. Remember, a small percentage of a big number is a big number! And of course, the harms of covid extend well beyond initial infection. Long covid is real and affects kids. Even mild infection leads to missed school, family stress, and takes away from the more normal life that we've worked so hard to restore to our children.

These risks are worth preventing, and we know that covid vaccines prevent them. Data from literally billions of people around the globe has shown that these vaccines are incredibly effective. In addition to providing protection against infection and transmission, we've seen an unprecedented ability to prevent serious disease and death. Safety data has been similarly impressive, and any source claiming that the potential harms outweigh the benefits has simply not done any actual research. All this is true for kids, too. Data continues to emerge, and by the time you read this we will have even more robust evidence for the safety of pediatric covid vaccines. Reports of rare incidences that make splashy headlines—I'm looking at you, a very unhelpful, unscientific, unnuanced discussion of myocarditis—miss the mark. It's important to stay vigilant and to react quickly to any red flags, which is exactly what we've done. Adjusting schedules based on the risk of certain reactions (or choosing a different vaccine type, thank goodness there are so many options!) is something we expect. But it doesn't change the fact that the risks of vaccination are miniscule compared to the risks of covid. I've seen exactly zero cases of vaccine-induced myocarditis, and all reported cases have been treatable. I've seen *many* cases, on the other hand, of covid-induced myocarditis, including older children who spent weeks on life support and even a teenager who passed away.

The data will keep emerging, the science will keep evolving. I'm here for it. I've learned plenty of hard-earned lessons during this pandemic, and an important one has been just how little we've told parents about the limited evidence we have in pediatric medicine. It's a real issue (and a particular pitfall of "data-driven parenting") that leaves pediatricians using a lot of common sense, biology, and clinical expertise to decide how to help you keep your kids healthy. So I'm truly excited to see so much research being done, so much focus on how to safely and effectively protect kids from covid. And the evidence we have at this point is so much more than we have for a huge number of treatments that we give to kids every day!

It's certainly infinitely more extensive and robust than the science we have behind any vitamin, supplement, pill, or medication that we use to treat covid (and a variety of other conditions) in kids. The anti-vaccine propaganda machine has made it all too easy to think we should deny children the protection they deserve from a highly studied vaccine, usually in order to sell whatever highly unstudied remedy they are trying to peddle instead. It's okay to just say no, to refuse to get caught up in the unscientific hype. Covid is here to stay. The choice is between covid infection and vaccination, and the choice is crystal clear.

Same for the seasonal flu shot. The decision to get your yearly influenza protection—for your children, yourself, and all caretakers—can be a similarly unagonizing one. We have decades more data to support just how safe this vaccine is for kids. Combine that with centuries of evidence that shows the devastating and deadly impact of flu in children (especially infants) and you'll quickly understand why I view this seasonal shot as just another crucial component of the routine childhood immunization series. No need to waste precious parental energy in an internal debate. Feel free to follow my lead, jump with joy when the flu shot becomes available every fall, and line the whole family up to get their dose of influenza protection.

THE BOTTOM LINE

5 out of 5 Pediatrician Parents Agree

1. "Natural" is *not* always better—it's not always even different! The divide between "natural" and "chemical" is arbitrary. Our bodies handle the active ingredients from so-called supplements exactly the same as they handle a synthesized compound with that same active ingredient.

2. Anything that you put in your (or your child's) body is medicine. By definition, if you are taking something to see an effect, that makes it a medicine—and all medications have side effects. Make sure the problem you're treating is worth giving medicine for, and that you chat with your pediatrician about potential risks, before trying any supplement.

3. Vaccines are tragically the greatest victim of the "natural is better" naturalistic fallacy. It's why anti-vaccine rhetoric has existed since the invention of vaccines. Predatory propagandists, who use the internet to trade immunization lies for power and profit, however, are new. And they orchestrate every anti-vaccine lie you'll find.

4. All vaccine fearmongering is easily debunked. The biggest myths— that vaccines cause autism, that the ingredients are unsafe, or that spacing out vaccines is a good idea—are patently untrue.

5. It's never too late to vaccinate! If you've been hesitant to protect your child with some, or even all vaccines, it's still worth catching up. Pediatricians are delighted that you've found information to empower your immunization decision and will happily work with you to get your little one back on track.

6. All vaccines are life-saving. I personally opt into every available immunization, including flu and covid vaccines for my whole family. I counsel all parents to do the same and feel confident in this choice.

CHAPTER 12

PLAY IT SAFE

Keeping Safety—and Fun!—
Front and Center as Your Child
Explores Free Play

In a world of mounting parental anxiety, it's harder than ever to know what you should actually worry about. Helicopter parenting is so 2004, and #SnowplowParenting, where parents push all obstacles out of the way, was trending for all the wrong reasons. But how do you balance safety with permissive play? If you're like me, the idea of total "free-range parenting," where toddlers go solo rock climbing and "supervision" is a dirty word, holds no appeal. The idea, though, that allowing for self-guided exploration, and some of the cuts and bruises that it inevitably brings, is important for your little one's development and protective against anxiety makes a lot of sense.

Finding the balance between all-or-none helicopter and free-range parenting is an ongoing journey for me. It is for most parents, as our biggest, hardest task is to guide our children through this world as safely as possible yet still give room for them to build autonomy. There is, as always, no single right answer. Moderation is a good mantra, and striving toward a middle ground between helicopter and free-range extremes makes sense for most. How much you push yourself in either direction will depend on your own personality (hello from an anxious mother with helicopter instincts!), your child's response, and your parenting style. Each decision is a moment in time, and part of a bigger picture.

It's true that you can just "figure it out," follow your instincts, and feel empowered to make risk assessments as daily activities arise. But you can also do a little planning and set yourself up for success.

During the peak of the pandemic and into the following years, as children continued to be deprioritized when it came to preventing covid infection, the topic of risk came up a lot. I reflected on it daily and answered hundreds of questions. We parents felt trapped, forced to accept risks that weren't fair for our children, expose them to covid because the harms of continuing to isolate were too great. It felt unique to that moment, a new dilemma of risk acceptance forcing us to make seemingly impossible choices. But the reality was that this wasn't anything new. While I would never minimize the fact that this situation was a failure of our society to protect children, being forced to accept the risk of harm to our children, preventable or not, is an inevitability. This realization helped me make decisions, counsel parents, and choose the option that best balanced risk of exposure from risk of isolation. It also helped me apply this same framework to other daily choices. I realized, concretely, why free-range toddler rock climbing held no appeal: What is the proven benefit of this level of risk-taking that you wouldn't get from laid-back playground exploration? I doubled down on my own mindfulness, working on my own anxiety and risk acceptance and trusting that I would make the choices that made the most sense for my family.

I also came to a new level of acceptance about the world around me. I would try to advocate for change, push policy that protects kids from the very preventable harms they face in this increasingly unstable world around us. But on a day-to-day level, I knew there would be many risks I couldn't control. And then, another light bulb—what *could* I control? I could decide which situations I allowed my child to find herself in, which places she would be allowed to explore. I could work to maximize the safety in those places—both indoors and outdoors—and then strengthen my efforts to take a step back and truly let her play.

This realization and reflection prompted a shift. I focused on the measures I could take to make her environment safer and minimize the chances of harm. I poured the most energy into serious harms, forcing myself to accept and expect bumps and scrapes. I set my child up for the safest play possible, so that I could promote the freest play possible.

Finding your version of safe, free play isn't always easy, but it starts with some simple steps. There are plenty of concrete ways to remove big dangers from indoor and outdoor adventures. So let's go through them, starting with the "toddler-proofing" basics that make it easier to engage in low-stress indoor play.

Safety First

Here are a few basics on how to toddler-proof your home.

1. Get those gates.

Stairs are a common, and frequently preventable, source of toddler injuries. If your home has stairs, it's a good idea to secure gates before your little one starts to crawl, glide, walk, run, and eventually catapult themselves toward this specific danger. And steer clear of baby walkers. As we talked about in my first book, these devices don't help kids learn to walk and instead give unstable mobility that makes tumbles down stairways much more likely.

2. Do a quick home survey.

It's always good to do a quick home inspection from time to time, even if there aren't any little ones looking to explore the potential dangers of your living space. Take this opportunity, then, to do a quick review of your home's standard safety features. Locate your fire extinguisher, check smoke and carbon monoxide detectors, and secure any heavy, easily-toppled furniture to the wall—especially in rooms where your little one spends their time.

While you're perusing your home, you'll also notice any mechanical hazards you've left strewn about. It happens, and there's no judgment—my home is a mess, too. Specifically, you'll put away things like button batteries (or any batteries, really), small hardware (nuts, bolts, screws, etc.), and other assorted plastic or metal tiny objects. You don't have to over-stress, just take a day to find safe storage for these items that kids love to adventurously—and dangerously—put in their mouths.

3. Secure cleaning supplies.

A common, tragically underappreciated potential peril during the toddler years is ingestion. Kids eat anything at this age. Yes, it's ironic that your two-year-old will try drain cleaner before they try broccoli. But they will, and every-thing else. No need to stress. Just take the time to prep. Ingesting cleaning products, antifreeze, and other industrial liquids can have devastating effects. Long before the horror of Tide pod challenges, I witnessed all sorts of internal inju-ries from caustic ingestion, so put it all away, after every use, and secure the cabinet with a childproof lock.

4. Safely store medicines, vitamins, and supplements.

Same for medicines, vitamins, and supplements. Pills look like candy, and any medicinal treatment carries the potential for harm. There are a variety of tablets, tinctures, liquids, and powders that can cause a variety of damage—sometimes even life-threatening damage, and sometimes even with just a tiny amount ingested. Childproof bottles are great but aren't foolproof. Human error is real and the most attentive parents leave bottles open. Kids find ways to, intentionally or not, smash prescriptions open. Your days of medications on nightstands are over, a small inconvenience that I promise is worthwhile. Secure everything just like you did with cleaning supplies and remember those pain relievers you keep in your bag count too (stashing my whole purse in the same kitchen cabinet I stored meds became a quirky habit of mine). Rules apply to your guests as well. One day, I remembered just how much I loved my friend when she came to visit me and my toddler, promptly told me there was ibuprofen in her purse, zipped it up and asked where she could safely store it.

5. *Be smart about firearms.*

It's not political, and it's not judgmental. It's also not an opinion: firearms are the leading cause of death in children. And many of these deaths are accidents. If you have firearms in the home, they need to be stored securely with a childproof lock and with the ammunition separate. No exceptions. It's also completely okay to ask parents how any possible guns they have in the home are secured before your kid goes over for a playdate.

6. *Refresh your resuscitation skills.*

It's great to stay up to date with basic resuscitation skills like CPR and the Heimlich maneuver, whether or not you have kids. And as kids grow, the techniques change a bit, making a review course all the more useful.

WTF, Monkeypox? When Infectious Outbreaks Won't Give You a Break

The year was 2017, a time that feels as if it existed approximately fifty years before the post-covid era. As a new parent, and a highly anxious one, I was keenly aware of the seemingly endless infections that the outside world held for my daughter—and by extension, that visitors could bring into my home. Covid didn't exist, but I was still worried; RSV, flu outbreaks, and a host of other respiratory viruses threatened to enter our home and land my daughter in the hospital.

My anxiety was founded in reality but certainly disproportionate. But the truth is, when it comes to infants, especially newborns, everyday colds carry a bigger risk. It makes sense to be more cautious when deciding how much infectious exposure makes sense. This is why I limit exposure as much as possible during the first month of life and loosen up my restrictions gradually (check out my first book's very long, detailed, scientific chapter on this topic!).

Your baby is a toddler now. Their lungs are more mature, their immune systems better able to stave off viral intruders—or, at the very least, more of the serious harms they can wreak. There's still a real risk, however, of getting sick and even needing the hospital for cold viruses (including but not limited to flu, RSV, and covid) for babies and toddlers compared to older kids and adults. It's more than reasonable to want to protect your little one from as much disease and suffering as possible! In a society that has politicized public health, there's more unhelpful, unnuanced advice than ever. If you look online, it seems that there are only extremes: accept all risks and welcome infection into your home with open arms, or let fear of disease dictate your entire social calendar.

Extremes are never the answer. They also aren't necessary in this case. There are plenty of ways to continue to minimize the risk of contagious illnesses while accepting the fact that they won't be completely preventable. There will be cases where, even amid whatever viral surge du jour surrounds you, the benefits of childcare, school, and hosting a special visitor outweigh the risks. Other times, the infections around you will be reason enough to modify your routine, if you can, and minimize exposure.

You'll make the decisions that best align with the unique risk/benefit balance for your family and take it day by day. And whatever you decide, you should feel empowered to set the limits that work for you. When I do welcome visitors during viral surges, I frequently keep my newborn rule and have a VIP-only invite list. Here are some other strategies that can help you set boundaries when welcoming these special guests.

- No sick or recently sick visitors need to urgently cuddle or be close to your little one.
- You should feel empowered to require proof of vaccination for all childhood immunizations, flu shot, whooping cough booster, RSV shot (for those eligible), and covid vaccine before allowing anyone to be in close contact with your child.
- Handwashing is key. Have visitors wash their hands when coming inside and also sanitize or wash hands before holding or playing with your little one.
- Masks are a great tool, and not just for covid! They are extremely effective at preventing RSV and flu transmission, as well as the other viruses that cause serious illness in babies and toddlers. It's totally fine to ask visitors to wear a mask in your home, or when near your little one, or when holding them, or some combination of these.
- No one needs to kiss a baby or toddler, especially if it's not a primary caregiver. Feel free to tell any well-intentioned friend or relative that the pediatrician prescribes a smooch-free visit!

The Great Outdoors

Taking time to stay active, enjoy nature's beauty, and bask in the joy of unbridled outdoor play is more important than ever in today's turbulent, stressful world. Yet the physical dangers of venturing outside of your home are real. Of course, the online parenting chorus of conflicting advice makes it seem impossible to even protect your child from sun, water, and bugs without somehow imperiling your child in ways you didn't even think to worry about. Never fear, there truly are safe and effective ways to enjoy outdoor play with minimal risk.

Sun day, fun day

Playing in the sunshine is a crucial part of childhood—as long as you remember that all kids need sun protection before heading outdoors. Even on cloudy days, or when the temperature drops, there can be more sun exposure than you might think. However, it's easy to get caught up in the online stress over sunscreens, sunburns, "chemicals" on skin and feel overwhelmed by something as simple as free outdoor play. Let's take a step back and remember that playing outdoors is meant to be fun—and it's super important for child development. Ditch the hot takes and #ads, follow these rules, and go have a good time!

1. Seek shade.

Some sun exposure is unavoidable. No need to become an outdoor vampire; just schedule some breaks from direct sun and choose shady areas for rest and play when possible. I like to put toys and outdoor pools in shaded corners, and take out-of-the-sun hydration breaks to beat the sun and the heat.

2. *Cover up. A lot.*

Toddler bikinis are out. If you get any traditional bathing suits that leave way too much skin exposed as gifts, save them for some quick photo shoots. Then get yourself some real summer gear in the form of UV-ray-repelling rash guards, zip-up suits, and water shirts. Our hot-weather uniform was a one-piece, long-sleeve zip-up water suit. Sometimes my daughter rocked "boy" bathing suit bottoms and a long-sleeve rash guard. I often put her in these outfits even if swimming wasn't on the schedule—playground sprinklers frequently made waterproof gear a plus, and the UV protection was enough to make it worthwhile no matter what. Hats were also mandatory as an added layer of facial protection (in addition to sunscreen, of course). Yes, I'm the mom who made my child wear her waterproof hat all day on the beach. There was a lot of luck involved, but in the end I'm proud of the results: I can report that as a result of this technique, combined with head-to-toe sunblock, my daughter has never had a sunburn.

3. *Make SPF your BFF.*

There's needless anxiety around the topic of sunscreen, and if you are ready to shut out the noise and embrace science and safety, here's the quick and dirty. All humans, including all children, need head-to-toe sunblock on any exposed skin before spending time outdoors. It's not a debate, and it's one of the clearest benefit-outweighs-any-potential-risk situations we have when it comes to parenting decisions. UV rays are carcinogens. They cause cancer. They can trigger and worsen a host of medical conditions as well. And they cause cancer.

The sun causes cancer. That's all you need to know. We have decades of randomized controlled trials with long-term follow-up showing that sunscreen use decreases the risk of skin cancers (namely squamous cell carcinoma, basal cell carcinoma, and melanoma). Unfiltered UV rays have exactly zero health benefit. You will get identical mood benefits from sunscreen-filtered sunlight. If vitamin D deficiency is an issue, your pediatrician will address it with a safe, convenient, and often gummy-delicious supplement. Anyone suggesting that you ditch UV protection is, intentionally or not, promoting a decision that could give your child cancer.

Whichever sunscreen best stays on your child's skin (choose SPF 30 or higher to assure adequate protection) is the right one. I avoid sprays that can disperse in the wind and leave gaps even with expert application. Today's sunscreens can technically last up to eight hours after a single application, but with water play and everyday sweating it's great to reapply more frequently (pediatric dermatologists recommend staying on an every two hour reapplication schedule). It's really that simple. Feel free to skip the rest of this section and move on if that closes the case for you!

A quick word on the "chemical" sunscreen panic: If you're fretting over "mineral" versus "chemical" sunscreens, you're not alone. Don't worry, I've got you covered. Here's the nit-ty-gritty of sunscreen selection that will de-stress making your summer shopping list.

There are two ways that sunscreens can block UV rays: by using "mineral," also known as "physical" filters, or using "chemical," also known as "organic" filters. Mineral filters, like titanium dioxide and zinc oxide, work by refracting ultravio-let radiation away from the skin—i.e., they physically block UV rays. Mineral sunscreens aren't absorbed into the skin, and in the past this meant that they were an aesthetically unappealing choice (think of the '90s prototypical lifeguard with a whistle around their neck and bright-white paste on their nose). People tended to like them less, and even apply too little in order to avoid this patented look. But advances in micronization of filters has changed the game, and you can readily find cosmetically acceptable options these days.

"Chemical" filters are actually "organic" materials made from aromatic compounds (like oxybenzone, avobenzone, octocrylene, and ecamsule), which absorb UV radiation. Interestingly enough, it turns out that "physical" filters also do this in addition to their job of "refracting," blurring the line between chemical and mineral when it comes to the chemistry behind them. Indulge me in a thought exer-cise: How might you have reacted differently to "chemical" sunscreens if they had instead, consistently been called "organic" sunscreens? It would be just as accurate to talk about "organic" and "inorganic" sunscreens, and we might be primed to worry more about the "inorganic" option in that case! There's no need to stress either way, but it's a good reminder of the naturalistic fallacy.

People love to use chemophobia, the totally normal but totally counterproductive instinct to fear "chemicals," to sell leafy-green labeled "natural" products. So let's stick to the science and talk about the actual risks. Chemical sunscreens are absorbed in very small quantities into the bloodstream. This leads to a bunch of theoretical risks but not a lot of real world ones. Remember, the dose makes the poison, and most people will never see enough systemic sunscreen to have any biologically plausible effect. Low-quality evidence, primarily in animal models, suggests there *could* be hormonal effects. It's not compelling data, but it signals a possibility and the need for ongoing research.

If the evidence is so shaky, why do we see some countries restricting the use of chemical sunscreens? Don't get it twisted—it has *nothing* to do with risk from human absorption. Instead, it's an important but separate ecological issue. Some ultraviolet filters have been found in the tissues of fish species, raising concern for downstream environmental impact (for example, oxybenzone affects coral reef larvae and may be related to coral reef bleaching). It's a complex issue involving public health, biology, and a greater understanding of interconnected ecological systems than I can fully understand, let alone explain here.

Where does that leave you? Exactly where you started: choosing the sunscreen that fits your family's needs. The priority is a high-SPF lotion that gets on and stays on your child's skin. If chemical filters give you personal or environmental anxiety, don't let them—there's a great alternative! When applied properly, mineral sunscreens are just as effective (if not more effective), so feel free to make them your go-to option. It's time for another reminder that there's no "safe" or "unsafe" in life, or with any parenting decisions. There's just the risk of doing something compared to the risk of not doing that thing. If mineral sunscreens didn't exist, it would be a no-brainer to embrace the chemical option. It's why, when I forgot to bring sunblock and someone offered theirs to me and my daughter, I slathered it on us without looking at the ingredients. If "chemical" options are easier to apply, work better with your child's skin, or just make sense for your family for whatever reason, that's great, too.

Water safety

When it comes to water safety, I'm definitely "extra." But it's a case where my anxiety does have real data behind it: drownings remain a leading cause of death in the toddler years. It makes sense to be thorough and take all possible measures to prevent them.

You don't have to indulge anxiety, but you do have to set some firm water-safety rules. There's no "safe" depth of water, and the saying that kids can drown in an inch of water is true. So treat all bodies of water the same: kiddie pools, bathtubs, basins all dictate the same supervision as lakes and oceans. This means you'll always watch attentively, and always stay physically close (no more than an arm's length away is a good rule). Swim toys and floaties are fine, but don't change my level of supervision.

As kids learn to swim, the arm's-length rule will of course change. But supervision doesn't. I'll die on the hill that everyone, even confident adult swimmers, needs a swim-time buddy. I'm also a fan of teaching kids how to swim as early as possible, recognizing that, like everything else, this is a question of privilege. Financial and logistical barriers make access to pools, bays, lakes—let alone swim lessons—challenging. Do your best, and however/whenever you teach your kid to swim is totally great.

Insect protection

Last, but not least, on our list of outdoor safety strategies is how to protect your little one from creepy crawlies—and, most important, from the bites and infections they bring along for the ride.

1. Use physical barriers.

You can start your anti-bug crusade by placing a few simple, effective barriers around your child. Screens on windows and doors, kept in good repair, are a great first step. Most outdoor play tents and strollers come with mesh netting that you can keep closed to block out bugs. Dressing in long sleeves and pants (with shirts tucked into pants and pants tucked into socks for even more protection) and wearing closed shoes is another helpful strategy. Light colored clothing tends to attract fewer mosquitos and makes it easier to see and remove ticks.

2. You'll need bug spray, at least sometimes.

I grew up in the Connecticut woods, not too far from a spirochete-inspiring, eponymous town called Lyme. The deer tick was almost always on our minds, and we routinely performed head-to-toe skin checks after every outdoor play session. Each summer day ended with a full body inspection, during which we gingerly removed any attached ticks, saved and sent them to be identified, and checked with our doctors to see if any prophylactic meds were needed. It was a necessary precaution. I've had friends and family members battle not only Lyme, but its cousins anaplasmosis and ehrlichiosis. This tiny pest is really no joke.

Again, there's no need to lose sleep over bug-related anxiety. The only reason to bring up the fact that ticks (and mosquitoes) carry serious diseases is because—all together now—the internet is trying to convince you that protecting your child from these illnesses is an impossible task. The same chemophobia that turns parents away from cancer-preventing sunscreen is also used to create needless bug repellent panic. But before we can dive into the details, we have to take a step back. Just like with sunscreen, bug spray exists for a reason. We aren't putting it on our kids for fun (as their toddler screams of protest will confirm). And while the benefit of not scratching itchy bites all summer is a real one, it's just the tip of the iceberg. Mosquito and tick-borne illnesses are serious. They cause devastating morbidity and mortality around the world. It's not just malaria, it's not just Lyme disease. There's a whole microscopic world of nasty organisms that, miraculously enough, you can protect your child from with simple, readily available sprays.

You should feel empowered to use insect repellents whenever your child is likely to be exposed to ticks and/or mosquitoes. Conversations about environmental impact and the (again, mostly theoretical) risks from systemic absorption are complicated. If you want to take a deeper dive, I've got the info for you here. If you want to trust that all registered repellents meet strict standards for toxicity and safety, based on an EPA protocol to minimize potential hazards to humans, that's great as well.

Here's a quick look at the commonly available "synthetic" (DEET, icaridin, IR3535) and "non-synthetic" repellents you're most likely to find, especially in the United States.

YOUR DEET-AILED GUIDE TO THE MOST COMMON INSECT REPELLENTS

DEET

What makes it great: DEET (chemical name N,N-diethyl-meta-tolu-amide) is the oldest, most effective repellent in common use. It's efficient, long-lasting, and protects against both ticks and mosquitoes.

Who can use it: DEET is approved for use in kids over two months of age. The theoretical risk from systemic absorption (see the next paragraph) has led some to recommend against using DEET when pregnant. It's not a universal recommendation. The environmental protection agency, for example, thinks it's just as safe in pregnancy as the alternatives. Now that there are likely safer and equally effective alternatives, I'm fine with the advice to use mostly DEET-free products during pregnancy. But please don't stress if you come into contact with DEET-containing products (or even use it from time to time) when pregnant.

Potential harms: When people ingest DEET or are exposed to it at intentionally harmful levels, it can cause brain toxicity including seizures and even coma. But with routine exposure, the only real danger is skin or eye irritation.

DEET can be absorbed into the bloodstream if it's directly sprayed onto the skin. The risks from this type of exposure are theoretical, with no evidence of any proven or specific effect. Animal studies have been largely reassuring, and while lab rats can have heart, breathing, and brain issues with chronic doses, this is unlikely to translate into issues for typical human application. Reassuringly, these DEET-exposed rats don't seem to have any reproductive or developmental problems.

DEET gets a lot of flak when it comes to environmental impact. As is usually the case, it's a very complex topic. The TL;DR is that DEET that's used on human skin has been found in surface and groundwater, posing an incompletely understood risk to aquatic species. Some data points to feeding issues in caddis flies, developmental issues in harlequin flies, respiration problems in algae, anemia in carp, and movement issues in cockroaches. There's a larger ecological discussion that's warranted, and that you may decide to consider in your assessment of personal risk versus benefit.

The final downside of DEET is cosmetic: it can damage clothing, plastics, acrylics, and more, so be careful where you spray.

Icaridin/picaridin

What makes it great: Icaridin is similar to DEET in a lot of ways, namely in its effectiveness in repelling ticks and mosquitoes. Unlike DEET, however, it's odorless, nongreasy, and doesn't degrade plastic or acrylic. It's generally less irritating than DEET but can cause some eye and skin irritation. Icaridin evaporates more slowly from the skin, so some posit that it may have a longer lasting repellent action than DEET.

Who can use it: Formulations of up to 10 percent icaridin or picaridin are safe to use in children over six months and often a preferred repellent for pregnant people. While we don't have a ton of pediatric or pregnancy data, the data we have is reassuring. We also know that absorption from the skin to the bloodstream seems to be much less with icaridin/picaridin than DEET. This means that any theoretical, systemic effects should be even less likely—making systemic effects with typical use less likely, too.

Potential harms: Data continues to emerge, but the studies we have now suggest that there aren't any serious environmental harms from typical use of icaridin/picaridin. As with DEET, it's a complex, evolving ecological conversation. Large doses have been toxic to fish, but there doesn't seem to be a lot of water contamination. Icaridin/picaridin can bind to the soil but tends not to travel much farther than that—and is nontoxic to the birds and land animals that come into contact with it. Animal studies have also been reassuring: lab rats exposed to icaridin/picaridin don't develop cancer, reproductive issues, or other serious health issues.

While not a real mark against it, I get frustrated with marketing icaridin as a "DEET-free" alternative. It's technically true, but still manipulative. The safety profiles of DEET and icaridin are pretty equivalent, and most consumers don't realize that "DEET-free" just refers to a synthetic compound more alike to DEET than it is different.

IR3535

What makes it great: IR3535 is one of the newest synthetic bug repellents on the market and tends to be the gentlest on skin. It has good protection against ticks and mosquitoes, is odorless, and has the best safety data if it's accidentally inhaled or ingested.

Who can use it: Like icaridin/picaridin, IR3535 is a favorite recommendation for pregnant people. It's also considered safe for children over six months.

Potential harms: There isn't a ton of downside with this one, and the side effect profile is generally better than both DEET and icaridin. This compound can cause eye irritation, but that's pretty hard to avoid for any product (most things can be irritating when they get in your eye!).

It's a newer product, meaning that there's less data. This might be why it seems safer—less time to do studies means less time to find problems. But the evidence available so far is compelling, suggesting that it's likely better tolerated and with less risk of serious harm in humans. The full environmental impact is even less clear than for DEET and icaridin/picaridin, but since so little seems to get into the surroundings, and based on the chemical properties of the compound, the potential for ecological effects is very low.

Non-synthetic repellents

Why they're great: Alternative to synthetic repellents, conveniently called "non-synthetics," are derived from essential oils. The most commonly used essential oils are lemon eucalyptus, citronella, andiroba, and neem-oil. Chemically, these oils are mixtures of volatile organic compounds–like monoterpene and sesquiterpene—that plants produce to defend themselves against predatory insects.

Who can use them: It really depends! Lemon eucalyptus oil is *not* safe for children under the age of three. Essential oils *can* be absorbed into the skin, and this risk is higher in babies and toddlers (who have a larger surface area compared to their body size). Kids are also much more likely to accidentally (or intentionally, especially with sweet smelling substances) put oil-covered skin in their mouth. These seemingly small quantities of swallowed oil add up, and can lead to a significant ingestion. All this means that the systemic risks of lemon eucalyptus oil specifically pose too much of a risk to young children to make them worth trying. When this compound gets into the bloodstream, it can cause serious stomach irritation, vomiting, breathing problems, brain changes, seizures, and even coma and death.

Other oils are usually considered to be okay if used correctly, although safety studies are very limited in the pediatric population.

Potential harms: One of the biggest downsides of non-synthetic repellents is their efficacy—it's bad. In practice, they are much, much less effective than the synthetics. Their volatility means they dissipate quickly and have a short time of action. Different oils also offer varying levels of protection against different insect species, and it tends to be a much narrower range of ticks and/or mosquitos that a particular compound can effectively repel.

Essential oils frequently leave greasy residues and stains, especially on clothing. More significantly, I've seen them trigger allergies, eczema, and can irritate sensitive skin (and eyes, of course, if they get in there). Non-synthetic doesn't mean "safe," and I've also seen an essential oil overdose in a toddler when they drank the sweet-smelling liquid!

Lemon eucalyptus oil is a total nonstarter for kids under three, but if you choose to use other oils for yourself or your child, make sure to use appropriately in small amounts on exposed skin. When you're done, keep them stored away alongside your other insect repellents to avoid any unintentional ingestion.

THE BOTTOM LINE

5 out of 5 Pediatrician Parents Agree

1. There is so much in this world we can't control, and parenting a toddler will always mean accepting risk. Focusing on the serious harms—and pouring energy into how to best mitigate them—will help you feel confident in allowing your child to explore the freest, safest play possible.

2. You can "toddler-proof" your home —or at least significantly decrease the risk of serious in-home injuries—with a few simple steps. Avoid baby walkers, put up gates securely at stairwells, survey your home's safety features, use secure locks to store medications and cleaning supplies, and make sure all firearms are locked away with childproof systems and with the ammunition separate.

3. You are allowed to set limits about the risks your child is exposed to—both inside and outside your home. You should never be made to feel bad when you ask about firearm storage before playdates. You can also feel empowered to restrict your child's socializing to non-viral, vaccinated individuals. Sick visitors can wait, it's okay to require proof of immunization, and basic hygiene (including masks when infectious risk is higher) is the name of the game.

4. It's cool to be obsessive when it comes to water safety. Drownings are a leading cause of death for toddlers. Your little one needs continuous supervision when in any body of water, even if it's only an inch deep (kiddie pools and shallow baths absolutely count!). Floaties and water wings are really just toys and don't change the supervision requirements for your little one.

5. Having fun in the sun is a normal, wonderful part of childhood. Don't let the stress take away the joy! You can embrace both free outdoor play and the measures that make it safer.

6. The sun is a carcinogen—UV rays cause cancer! Thank goodness we have safe, effective sunscreens that keep our kids safe. In addition to covering up exposed skin where possible and taking in sun in moderation, your child will need to use sunscreen consistently (you'll choose a mineral or chemical option based on your preference).

7. Protecting your miniature outdoor adventurer against insect bites is also worthwhile. Using screens, mesh, netting, and fuller-coverage clothing is a great first step. But there will still be cases where an insect repellent is necessary. Bug bites don't "just" cause miserable itching but carry a world of serious tick and mosquito-borne diseases! There are lots of DEET and DEET-free options, with the synthetic options being by far the most effective. If you consider essential oils, steer clear of lemon eucalyptus oil, the (counterintuitively) most dangerous insect repellent for children.

CHAPTER 13

BRAVE NEW WORLD

Navigating Hard Topics, Tough Questions, and Guiding Your Child Through an Ever-Changing World

"Mommy, when are you going to die?"

It was 8:00 p.m., and bedtime was running later than I would have liked for a school night. I was on clinical service, tired but fulfilled from my ongoing week seeing patients in the hospital. Tomorrow was another early morning and likely another long day. Not the best time for a question like this. I gave some reassurance, a big hug, and promised my daughter we would talk about it in detail the following day. She fell asleep quickly, and I spent the night reviewing my resources and planning our conversation. The following morning, she went off to school smiling, well-rested and didn't bring up the topic. I rolled out of bed, showered, kissed her goodbye, and ordered a Trenta-sized latte with two extra shots.

Questions about hard subjects never seem to come when you'd like them to. And some topics are so challenging that it never feels like there's a good time to tackle them. Take a deep breath and remember that you are a thoughtful, caring parent. Let's go through the strategies I use when approaching difficult discussions, empowering you to guide your toddler responsibly and lovingly through the complex world around them.

TBH—Challenging Conversations, Questions, and Topics

1. Everything's on the table.

When in doubt, talk it out. Gone are the days of repression and propriety—at least at home. It's tempting to defer conversations indefinitely or avoid "advanced" topics. But you're much better off tackling these tricky subjects head-on. It's always better for your kid to get the information directly from you (they're hearing it already from others, even at this tender age), and it's always better for you to have a window into their evolving thoughts and feelings. Addressing hot-button issues is a necessary part of parenting, helping you set the stage for how your child forms their identity and creating a safe homebase for them to do so.

2. Pauses are your friend.

When in doubt, wait it out. No need to respond right away. You can ask for more info, or just validate that it's a good question. My favorite trick when I draw a blank is to say that I need to think about how to explain my answer and plan to look up information and report back! Taking some time will give you the opportunity not only to get the info you need but to also reflect on your own reactions. You'll unpack any maladaptive internalized beliefs (hello, body image issues that I don't want to project onto my anatomy conversation!) as you create some key discussion points.

3. Seek out the experts. The real experts.

When you do your research, remember that not all "research" is created equal. When it comes to hot topics there's no shortage of bad takes. You can stay on track by focusing your energies on a few sources for each sticky subject. The content of your explanation is important but won't land how you want it to without the right delivery. It's why well-intentioned scripts from nonexperts that technically convey your point, but aren't geared to a child's developmental level, tend to be counterproductive. Instead, seek out credentialed experts, usually signaled with a background in child development and/or education, who have personal and professional expertise on a given subject.

For example, you'll learn the specific strategies to tackle your child's tough questions about racism not from me, a well-meaning white pediatrician, but from venerated antiracism educational professionals. These are the same resources that I relied on to reverse my own "color-blind" education (hey there, thirteen-year-old me watching *The Color of Friendship* after-school special). It's an ongoing journey that's challenging but worthwhile. There's the personal work of reframing racism as a systemic scourge rather than a series of "mean" actions, something that's been very liberating to me. It takes effort to keep engaging in this reflection, and even more hard work to play a role in dismantling societal institutions. But it takes a whole different type of skill to translate all of that reflection into language that my child can understand. We're fortunate to have access to great guides that break down conversations about race for children and adults alike. These guides encourage curiosity, allowing children to explore differences (including skin color) while embracing diversity and recognizing that unfair treatment exists. You'll pick up strategies to incorporate antiracist play into everyday life, learning that it's a journey, not a hashtag. Stressful discussions will undoubtedly arise, but the overarching experience should, and can, be positive.

You'll want to seek similar, developmentally geared, high-quality guidance for any and all other tough questions your child asks. Want to get ahead? You'll undoubtedly be asked questions—or want to proactively start a discussion—about bodies, anatomy, sexuality, gender, and consent. And just like taxes, death is guaranteed. As are a toddler's questions about it, usually when a parent is at their most tired and least prepared.

4. Stay honest—in a developmentally appropriate way.

I found my own approach to tackling tough questions through a lot of expert research, plenty of trial and error, and focusing on a few principles. The first policy is honesty. During the pandemic, I spent a great deal of emotional effort trying to embrace uncertainty without losing hope and learning to accept risk without minimizing reality. The struggle to bask in life's joys while understanding just how fleeting they may be (a.k.a. the human condition) is something I want to help my daughter tackle head-on.

Embracing reality means that I try my best to stay truthful in my answers to questions, even when I know it could be upsetting. As an example, I've never referred to death as "sleeping," and when my toddler asked me one day if dead people ever came back to life, I answered no. Of course, my phrasing was different, and choosing honesty doesn't mean ditching solace. I'm also a pediatrician with an appreciation for child development, and I'm a sensitive, loving mother who still wants to protect my child when I can. I deliver every harsh truth in developmentally appropriate terms, sharing only necessary information, and providing plenty of comfort. "Yes, Mommy will die like all people. I don't expect that will happen for a very, very long time. I love you [*big hug*], and we are safe. It's okay to worry about dying. I get sad and nervous sometimes when I think about dying, too. I'm usually busy being happy with you and Daddy and try to spend more time thinking about that. I'm always here if you have questions or need more hugs."

5. *Stay curious.*

It's all too easy to make assumptions, even when we don't realize we're making them. When it comes to these types of conversations, I found that I often assigned—and usually misassigned—intention to my daughter's questions. Maybe your child asks you about their friend's skin color, and you instinctively worry it's connected to discrimination. Or maybe you project your own fears onto them and confuse a matter-of-fact question about death with anxiety. Maybe it's simply an automatic assumption about motivation—you think you know why your little one wants an answer, but you haven't really dug into it. So dig in!

Curiosity is king. Encourage their question-asking, and ask your own. As parents, it's easy to feel like we need to have all the answers—or know where to get them. You'll do your research and give as much high-quality information as you can. But you also get to be curious and embrace uncertainty. It's a discussion, not a lecture. You'll get some useful context—"That's an interesting question, what made you think of that?" "Did someone say that in school? I'd love to hear more"—while modeling bidirectional learning.

Ch-ch-ch-ch-changes: Adjusting to New Siblings, Life Transitions, Social Stressors, and Beyond

Turn and face the strange: not just lyrics from one of my all-time favorite songs, but a fundamental truism. Even before the certain uncertainty of pandemic parenting, I learned quickly that change is a constant—so why not embrace it?

Even with the best planning, change is *hard*. You can't prevent all the stress it brings, but you can use these strategies to make life's seemingly endless transitions a little smoother for you and your toddler alike.

1. Talk about feelings and challenges.

A dozen chapters have gone by, giving you lots of time to incorporate your emotional-regulation modeling into your everyday routine. This includes talking about feelings and normalizing all sorts of negative emotions. Get ready to reap the benefits. When children have the vocabulary to name feelings—and feel empowered to talk about them openly—it's easier to get through them. And while you're basking in the skills you've refined from our earlier chapter on toddler behavioral regulation, take a minute to review the other strategies (visual schedules, pretend play, and so much more!) that you can use during these tough times.

2. Avoid surprises.

There's no right answer for when is the "best" time to tell your toddler a big change is about to happen. There will be a lot to consider developmentally. Most two-year-olds live on a day-to-day basis and can't think much beyond a week ahead. It makes sense when you think about how they only fully remember months of being alive! This means most toddlers will stress needlessly if you tell them about a big move to another state months and months before it happens. But giving a real heads-up—especially as they watch you take all the preparatory steps and start piecing things (anxiously) together by themselves—is key.

3. Get everyone on the same page.

Here's another throwback to our emotional regulation discussion: be deliberate and keep all messengers on the same page. When a change is on deck for your toddler, decide who you want to be the one to break the news (generally this should be you). Get all caretakers on the same page to make sure no one spills the beans early. Once the cat is out of the bag, you can let caregivers know how you've been framing the conversation so they can keep the message consistent.

4. Listen, listen, listen.

Another theme that I'm sure you've picked up on is that concerns are not always what they seem. It's easy to assume we know what's worrying our little one. A new sibling will steal attention! They'll miss their friends when you move out of state! It seems obvious, and we tend not to question our assigned motivation. But you'd be surprised. So go ahead and ask. And remember to listen. They might not tell you their truest, deepest worry right away, so be patient and keep an open dialogue.

5. Keep it real.

As a sensitive, worried human, my instinct is to lean a little too hard into positives. I'm constantly trying to reassure myself—and my daughter—that everything will be okay. The instinct to soothe is natural and helpful. Just be mindful that the urge to focus on the pluses of a situation isn't pushing away reality. I struggled not to follow every piece of difficult news with a qualifier—"Yes, we're moving, but you'll get this cool bedroom, want to see a picture?" Instead, I found it worked better to take that pause and acknowledge that change can really suck. "Moving is hard, and I know you'll miss your friends—I'll miss them, too!" It's okay to let your little one sit with that truth for a moment. It really is a growth opportunity, and it's incredibly validating. Embracing reality doesn't mean ditching comfort, and you'll still be able to hug, reassure, and provide the love and security they need.

6. Embrace resilience—both yours and your toddler's.

Toddlers are resilient. They deal with a lack of control and battle endless change daily. Big transitions are a stressful rite of passage. Provide support and take solace in their strength.

It's okay to have faith that both of you can handle whatever life sends your way.

Oh, Hello There, Interloper: Some Specific Tips for Welcoming a New Sibling

There's no limit to the various life transitions that can throw you and your toddler for a loop. It would be impossible to go through them all here, and I'm not even tempted to try. But I do want to explore one specific transition—getting a new sibling—and share a few pediatrician parent pro tips on how to help welcome your new addition.

Bringing another child into your family will be a time of transition—with plenty of older sibling emotions, behavioral changes, and a good dose of stress for everyone—no matter what. But there are definitely ways to make it less painful for everyone. The pediatrician parents I know generally favor trying to meet the new baby at home, not at the hospital, where your older child will feel more comfortable, see you in a familiar setting, and have a bit of a "home field" advantage. We also are big fans of having a small gift "from the new baby" on hand, and having one parent go inside first without baby to greet and prepare.

Jealousy is inevitable, but strategies that put an older sibling's needs first when it's so easy for them to become deprioritized with a much needier, more fragile baby go a long way. Newborn and toddler crying at the same time? Go to the toddler first. If the newborn is in a safe place, they'll be okay to cry for a few minutes, and big sib will feel cared for, remembered and protected, knowing that you are able to respond just as quickly as before a tiny intruder came to compete for their parent's attention. And all kids and adults—and especially toddlers—do best hearing yes instead of no. Thinking ahead of some age-appropriate expressions of love and "helpful" tasks for your older child (handing you wipes for diaper changes, caring for a doll or stuffed animal in parallel, giving the baby kisses on the toe rather than face) will help diffuse the inevitable tension.

THE BOTTOM LINE

5 out of 5 Pediatrician Parents Agree

1. Talking about hard topics is hard. But it's always better to address them preemptively and deliberately. You can get ahead of information before your little one hears it elsewhere—probably earlier than you think—and set the stage for open, honest, fact-based conversations that keep them happy and safe.

2. If you feel emotional, overwhelmed, or unsure how to answer a question—don't. Take a pause, then let your toddler know they've asked a smart, tricky question that will take some thought for you to answer. You can always let them know you'll be doing some research and reporting back later with an explanation.

3. Other ways to stay on track during challenging conversations are remembering to seek out talking points from the true experts, focusing on finding guidance that's both honest and developmentally appropriate, and encouraging curiosity (both your child's and your own!).

4. Keeping it real isn't mutually exclusive from providing comfort and a sense of safety. You can stay honest without sending your child into a spiral of existential angst. This can be accomplished by focusing on your individual child's concerns, staying attuned to developmentally appropriate language and concepts, and assuring as much love and security as possible.

5. Life transitions cause serious toddler stress no matter how much you prepare. There are ways to ease the pain, though. Validate the emotional turmoil your child is undoubtedly feeling, and don't assume you know what their biggest worries are. Mix up your coping strategies and the tools you share with your child.

Sometimes problem-solving makes sense, other times just listening to their concerns is the name of the game.

6. If your toddler is welcoming a new sibling, you can add specific strategies to your family's transition-tackling toolbox. Pediatrician parents generally favor meeting a new baby at home (not the hospital), having the "baby" give their older sibling a gift, checking on a crying toddler before a screaming newborn, and thinking of ways to include your toddler in caring for the adorable interloper they will, eventually, learn to love.

CHAPTER 14

LIVE AND LEARN

Fostering Your Toddler's Development However Your Style, Schedule, and Budget See Fit

Your child is a real person—moving, shaking, communicating, and more social than ever. Maybe you're watching them at home, maybe you have another caretaker, maybe they're in full-time daycare or have a scheduled playgroup. No matter what their day looks like, it's clear they are active and interactive, thriving as they explore the world around them.

Why, then, is your social media feed still filled with new, expensive toys that claim to be necessary in promoting your child's development? And why are you still getting ads for music classes and other activities hoping to trade your money for toddler education? Are they worth the effort and expense? What about that Montessori-inspired nursery that looks so beautiful on an influencer's grid no matter what filter they use? Should you trade in all your child's beloved toys and furniture for a new model that toddlers allegedly need for optimal development?

Each day, no matter how much your little one is crushing toddler life, you'll find more and more people trying to convince you that you're still not doing enough. However you spend your money is great—as long as it's what you want to do, and as long as you know what the actual benefit is. It's time to review toddler development, understand what they actually need (and don't need!) to meet their potential, and once again give you permission to simply *enjoy* playtime, no matter what it looks like.

Basics on Toddler Development

Just like with babies, the actual inputs that toddlers need to create an exploding neural network are quite simple. But the work those little brains are doing—and the skills they master in just a few years—are quite impressive. Developmental milestones, while still averages, are a helpful way to understand just how dramatically your (typically-developing) toddler's motor, social, and language skills will evolve. Their gross motor ability will go from crawling, scooting, or wobbly walking to running, climbing, and becoming coordinated enough to try some miniature athletics. In the fine motor domain, their basic grasp will develop into building block towers, pouring out of containers, and drawing scribbles, lines and even circles. Their language explosion is something to behold—a typical one-year-old who generally understands what people say but speaks a few (or no) words will grow into a three-year-old who communicates in full, mostly comprehensible sentences. Other cognitive skills blossom in an equally impressive way: toddlers master object permanence, a variety of problem-solving abilities, learn independence, become more social, imitate behavior, and start to grasp some abstract concepts.

Buy, Buy, Baby: Playtime Edition

One way that you'll get to witness these incredible gains is through your toddler's daily play. And their play is one of the main ways that they practice and master these skills. Play is, without a doubt, a super important part of child development. So does this mean that you must get your child that subscription for "development-promoting" toys? Do you need to overhaul your play space for a Montessori or other "research-based" design?

In short, no. All your toddler actually *needs* to grow and thrive is still a safe and interactive environment. It's something that can be built almost anywhere that there are loving people around them (and a few very bare-bones playthings). The specific toys or how they're laid out won't dramatically change your child's development. A toddler can thrive in any home that comes with spaces to explore and people to guide them through it.

There's a lot of hype behind specific makes and styles of toys, and there is certainly a good amount of profit-seeking behind baseless claims that tout a certain product as better than the next. But while brand worship doesn't make sense, the idea that some types of playthings—and how they're arranged in your home—will, on average, be more conducive to developmentally engaging play is a logical one. It's mostly common sense. It's not because there's a particular nursery feng shui that is scientifically proven to stimulate toddlers— it's just about how you facilitate play. If you have spaces where toys are accessible, *and* you encourage and allow for free play, it will be easier for your child to work on their motor, communication, and social skills on their own time.

As for specific toys, it's also key to keep the big picture in mind. More important than anything is *how* toys are used. A few examples: If your kid hates a toy (it happens!), or just doesn't use it a lot, there's no developmental benefit. If you find a toy, game, or book that *you* like, you'll be more likely to use it with them. Realizing that my three-year-old loved puzzles as much as I did was a (pun-intended) game changer, and spending $15 on a two-hundred-piece puzzle that we could do together was a no-brainer. Noisy electronic toys, on the other hand, often held her solo attention longer, and I kept some around for times that I needed a break. But the most obnoxious ones managed to get "lost" or "broken" (wink, wink) almost immediately, and I knew that they weren't necessary for any toddler "education."

If you're looking for some guidance on which playthings make sense for your toddler, there's nothing wrong with seeking out some recommendations! I've found it helpful to pivot from brand allegiance, though, and instead check in with my toddler's needs and wants when I look through reviews. One tool you can use when doing this is to focus on where they are in their play trajectory. All kids are different (I repeat, averages are averages and play preferences are highly individual), but you can anticipate how your child's play will progress using our understanding of typical development.

From around twelve to eighteen months, kids understand the purpose of toys and tend to use them as intended—a phone is a phone, a toy car is a toy car. They're mastering cause and effect, making games that let them practice learning this especially appealing (like mechanical cranks that make things pop out, peekaboo games, toys you can fill up and dump out, etc.). After this, from around eighteen to twenty-four months, is when pretend play steals the scene. As imagination develops, toddlers make inanimate objects carry out tasks (dolls eat play food, toy cars drive), and can even do some complex action sequences (the doll can eat, then go in the car, then be pushed across the room). Parallel play—engaging mostly with themselves alongside other children—is still more common than interactive play. In this phase, toddlers also love "extremes of movement," meaning swinging, climbing, and sliding start to hold enormous appeal. Toddlers expand upon and refine all these skills, especially pretend play, from age two to three years. Play scenarios become more complex, truly interactive, and social play is favored over solo play. Abstract concept mastery helps make play more creative: a block can now sub in as that pretend phone or toy car. More evolved motor skills bring new activities and games into the mix—throwing balls, riding tricycles, and playing some basic sports. By three to four years, imagination still dominates playtime, and is even more collaborative with other toddlers. Older toddlers can also participate better in group activities and really enjoy them—group singing, circle time, dance, and art classes become fast favorites.

The toys that let you confidently play with your child through all of these phases are the right ones. In the end, you'll know which playthings make sense for your child's personality, lifestyle, and your family's budget. Choosing "developmental" products is fine—they are often great! As a rule, these products require a higher level of engagement from your toddler if they actually want to have fun with them. For many parents, subscription boxes and specific-brands are a convenient way to fill a playroom. If that's the case, or if you simply like the aesthetics and have money to spare, go for it! Just remember that it's more than okay to embrace the toys you already have. Focusing on making a play space that's laid out according to your style and filled with whatever items you and your toddler enjoy most is what will set you up for success.

Nanny versus Daycare versus Neither: What's the Tea?

Just like there's no specific toy or game needed for vibrant, thriving toddler development, there's also no specific brand of childcare that's better or best. Any compassionate care-taker can create a world in which your child can explore the world around them. The specific activities are unimportant.

The only actual requirements to any daily schedule are: socializing with others; having space to crawl, cruise, walk, run and explore the world around them; hearing language and sounds; and having a few basic objects they can use in their blossoming world of imagination and parallel play. That's really it. Any reputable childcare center will provide these, and I can confidently say that there is no actual need for kids in daycare to engage in extracurriculars.

Taking a quick tangent away from development, it's time to address another frequent concern about daycare: getting sick. It is completely true that children in daycare will get sick a lot more, and it's common to have a toddler who's sick every few weeks (i.e., basically the whole winter) when they're in a childcare setting. It's miserable for parents, but it isn't harmful in the long term for kids. Whether they are exposed to viruses all at once, or over time, they'll have the same number of infections overall. Basic hygiene and up-to-date vaccines are all you need to optimize their health, and there won't be any immune system damage.

If you go the nanny/caretaker route—or stay home to care for the kids yourself—there's also no need to stress. Without the built-in socialization and enrichment of daycare, the pressure mounts higher to spend even more money on childhood "education." Yet the evidence shows that replacing a pricey toddler gym membership with a local library's worth of story time and free play in the children's section, as one example, is an excellent choice. Music, gym, yoga, and even math classes will provide the exact same developmental opportunities as any unstructured toddler get-together with age-appropriate toys and engaged caretakers. It's not that there's anything wrong with these activities! There are plenty of other potential benefits, including providing opportunities to socialize with other parents, or simply give a few scheduled hours between naps. If you want to spend that $30/hour on a toddler dance class, rock on! But you also should know that opting for (literally) free play will not doom your child to a life of educational disadvantage.

The less-is-more, play-is-enough approach to parenting really crystallized during the pandemic—for me personally and for countless other parents. The sudden onset of childcare closures, isolation, and a world of covid precautions made in-person, structured play less accessible than ever. Parents like me learned how incredibly resilient children are, and how they can absolutely reach their full potential without the enrichment activities we have become so used to. With daycare closed, and socialization initially limited, it was hard not to feel like the entire weight of my daughter's development rested on my shoulders. But I quickly saw how she was able to adapt, and how I was able to follow her lead. I recall one day of #stayathome parenting where we explored the outdoors together. It was remarkable to see her create her own learning experience through play, pointing to animals, plants, finding shapes and colors, and expanding her imagination. Did I know that some leaves are shaped just like stars? It's a particularly fond memory from a particularly dark time, and a reminder of the experiences one can find when structure and expectations loosen.

I also remind myself of the very real fact that traditional education is merely one way for children to grow and thrive. This is especially true for babies and toddlers. It wasn't until just a few decades ago that formalized curricula for preschoolers (let alone infants and toddlers) were the norm. To put it in perspective, just think of all of the certifiable geniuses out there who invented vaccines, cured diseases, created art and music, all after a childhood filled only with free play and without a single school class until the first grade!

THE BOTTOM LINE

5 out of 5 Pediatrician Parents Agree

1. Toddlers achieve a whirlwind of motor, social, cognitive, and language milestones in just a few years. It's impressive and amazing to witness! Play is one way they show off their skills, and a crucial way that they develop them.

2. There are endless ways to support your toddler as they progress through their stages of play and the world around them. Focus on laying out and filling your play space in whatever way makes you feel confident, and however facilitates your toddler's engagement.

3. When in doubt, keep it simple. There will be plenty of times where a noisy toy, gadget, or (*gasp*) even screen-based activities are needed to keep your child entertained. But most of the time, free play is best facilitated by the most basic playthings.

4. Kids in daycare get sick more frequently, earlier on, and it's miserable for parents. It's not dangerous, though, and it won't damage their immune system. Children who start school or childcare later eventually see all the same viruses.

5. There's no specific brand of childcare that's best for your child's development. Nanny, caretaker, daycare, preschool are all perfectly wonderful at this age, as long as they work for you and your lifestyle.

6. There's also no evidence that toddlers need formal education. Daycare curricula, toddler extracurriculars, and any structured activity is wonderful if it makes sense for your lifestyle and budget. But it's optional, and worth as much as the joy it brings your family.

CHAPTER 15

I SCREEN, YOU SCREEN, WE ALL STILL SCREEN

Why Screen Time Isn't Toddler Poison

The year was 2020. In the month of February, I felt like I was finally getting into my parenting groove. I was over a year into my new job as a fancy, grown-up "attending" doctor, and felt that maybe I did know what I was doing. After months of transition—new job, new state, new childcare, new commute, new life, new me—I had a stable routine. I started exercising, eating better, my toddler was sleeping through the night—is this what parenting really was like? My pregnancy and postpartum experiences had been grueling, and the second year had been filled with so much life stress. Could this be the turning point? Was I actually just nailing motherhood?

March 2020, as you already know, had other plans. As talk of the then novel coronavirus spread from whispers to screams, I put all my efforts into bracing myself as best as possible for the uncertainty to come. And as unprecedented times unfolded around us, I felt, like all parents, the waves and ripples of the pandemic expand into our daily life. To be a #PandemicParent was to just keep trying, and most pre-pandemic norms quickly and continuously evolved.

The most notable initial change was screen time. I had been practicing a moderation-based approach to TV watching since I already knew that there were plenty of times when the benefit to so-called "excessive" screen time outweighed any risk (naps on the couch while my daughter watched Baby Shark videos were a staple of my day-after-hospital-shift routine). Overall, my daughter's screen consumption approached official recommendations more often than not. But when COVID-19 hit New York City, all bets were off. I'm still grateful for the health, well-being, and support I maintained as a frontline worker. I was also able to arrange secure childcare earlier than most. And still, despite this much more normal routine than was typical for the time, we relied on screens. A *lot*. I quickly set aside any expectations—even my own modified, moderate expectations. I just had to get through, prioritize what was important to our big picture. I went into doctor mode and triaged the situation: Monitoring screen time could wait.

Since covid, it seems the world is starting to catch up to the privilege inherent in unrealistic screen time expectations. While the pandemic forced all parents to embrace "good-enough parenting," it was clear that the impossible challenges of working parenthood during a certifiable plague were not distributed equally. One day in July, as I doom-scrolled through social media, I stumbled upon a thread filled with blog posts and essays from parenting experts now compelled to repent their screen time abstinence-only ways. These parents were newly faced with the task of being the primary caretaker of their children (while working from home, of course, and without nannies or preschool to provide engagement and entertainment). It may not be March 2020, but there will always be cases where screen indulgence outweighs any risks, pandemic or none. The covid era crystallized even more to me that my realistic screen time counseling had always been the right approach.

As I explained in *Parent Like a Pediatrician,* screen time isn't baby poison--and it isn't toddler poison, either. Our desire to be judicious with screens comes from a good place. There *is* data to suggest that too much screen time—like anything—isn't a good thing. What exactly "too much" means, however, depends way more on your circumstance and how you balance the risks and benefits. And each decision, as always, is just for a moment in time.

We can be deliberate and do our best to keep screen use contained and balanced without succumbing to extremes. There's no need to pledge allegiance to arbitrary cutoffs or worry that thoughtful screen consumption will melt your child's brain. There's also no need to go back to the bad-old-days where unlimited screen binges were a child's norm (oh hey there, fourth-grade me watching One Saturday Morning and TGIF until my vision blurs). The answer is, of course, somewhere in the middle. It's time to pause, regroup, and review the commonsense principles that will guide your screen time use for your toddler—and for your whole family.

The 10 Screen Time Commandments, Toddler Edition

1. *Not all screens are created equal (some are inherently better than others).*

It's important to think about how screens are used and what content they can deliver, but some screens are just going to be better than others in almost any context. Trust your instincts. After years of restrictive guidelines, blog posts, and even outright shaming, it's all too easy to get caught in the trap that anything with a "screen" is automatically evil. For example, an interactive tablet designed for littles (V-Tech etc.) is much more like any other electronic toy than a fully functioning screen. A tablet that streams Netflix and YouTube videos, on the other hand, is basically a TV. It makes sense, but it's easy to get swept up in the hysteria. Playing with electronic toys, letting your toddler explore your e-reader (which is much more like a book than a true screen) or pressing on a touch-screen menu can essentially get free passes.

2. *Abstinence is impossible.*

We live in a world where screens—of all shapes and sizes— are omnipresent. Unless you go completely off the grid, there is a 100 percent chance your child will be around screens. It's much easier to control a child's screen exposure if you embrace it.

3. Less is more, but counting screen time minutes doesn't always make sense.

There's a reason we're even talking about screen time limits. A quick reminder: during my training, the world of official, pediatrician-sanctioned screen time recommendations was quickly evolving. Back in 2015, the sentiment was simple: screens are bad. The American Academy of Pediatrics recommended strict avoidance of visual contact with literally any type of screen (video chat, tablet-based activities, you name it) for kids under two years of age. Then suddenly, on a child's second birthday, they magically gained the mental capacity to handle up to two hours of screen contact every day. The backlash was expected and appropriate. With no compelling evidence to justify this restrictive approach, many pediatricians joined parents in asking the AAP to create realistic recommendations that acknowledged the complex science behind baby screen time. Previous, ultraconservative screen time guidelines were based on limited data, mostly observational studies whose design makes it very difficult to draw real conclusions. For example, a famous study linked sedentary behavior (including but not limited to watching screens) to childhood obesity. But, as always, correlation does not equal causation.

The associations we find are certainly multifactorial. As just one example, toddlers who watch TV programs with commercials for unhealthy food products could have an obesity risk increase simply due to this targeted advertising, rather than the duration of screen exposure. So after taking a hard look at the data (including new studies showing that video chat with family, intuitively, is important for social connection and actually provides more benefit than harm), the AAP did agree it was time to make some important—if small—changes. The new-and-improved 2016 AAP policy still bans solo, passive screen use until eighteen months, at which time parents may introduce no more than sixty minutes per day of "high-quality, educational" programming. But the key difference is that this recommendation doesn't include "constructive or connective" screens like video chatting, taking photos, making videos, looking at maps, or searching the internet to find information. These AAP rules were generally held as doctrine throughout my residency, and I'm grateful my training finished before the infamous 2019 WHO guidelines—suggesting a complete ban on screens for the first two years of life, followed by a strict sixty minutes per day limit from ages two to five years—came in place.

It certainly tracks that minimizing time with eyes glued to a screen will allow for all the important developmental activities a toddler needs. There is science, and it does support the idea that less is more. Young children who are exposed to screens beyond AAP recommendations have been shown to have differences in brain structure, changes in language development, and sleep. In 2023, for example, a study from Singapore showed that higher amounts of screen time use, reported by parents when their children were twelve months old, seemed to contribute to attention issues seen in those children nine years later.

The data is concerning, but it's also limited. The biggest problem with studying screen time is that it relies on observational data. It's extremely challenging to tease apart all the factors that may be contributing to the screen time–badness link. So many other factors are likely at play (absence of other developmental activities, access to early literacy, nutrition, socioeconomic status, just to name a few). Certainly, a good portion of the effects we see are because of these other associations. In the age of covid, we know now more than ever that a screen-free or limited-screen existence is a marker of privilege.

The other problem with using observational studies to support strict time cutoffs in screen recommendations is that most of them are designed the exact opposite way you'd want them to be. It's nothing that the researchers did wrong, it's simply another limitation of this type of study design. The only way to actually know what a "safe" amount of screen time is would be to take a bunch of babies and randomize them into groups where they get different daily screen exposures (zero minutes, twenty minutes, forty minutes, an hour, etc., etc.). This is, for obvious reasons, problematic and logistically challenging. It's hard from an ethical perspective to do a randomized trial and make a bunch of infants binge-watch Netflix while the others have a screen-free childhood filled with developmental activities. This means that our information relies on parents reporting how much screen time they allow kids to consume. Not only is this potentially inaccurate (I can't remember how much PBS Kids my daughter watched yesterday, let alone last week), but it also oversimplifies things. Current studies tend to divide children into two groups: those who consume more than the AAP recommended amount of screens, and those who don't. This means that those studies showing language delays, brain changes, and other screen-induced woes have had to group very different situations together. For example, an infant with four hours of TV time daily would be in the same category as one with twenty minutes of daily screen use.

In the end, the science is real, and there is data suggesting associations between screen use beyond AAP recommendations and developmental issues. Screen time moderation and cognizance is absolutely important. But the reality is that there is no magical time limit that will assure your child is free from the potential deleterious effects of screens. It's far more important to embrace all the other measures that help use screens in their appropriate and appropriately limited contexts, and focus less on tracking your kid's minute-by-minute screen consumption.

4. *The most, most important part of a screen is how it's used.*

There's an enormous difference between sitting a toddler in front of a tablet to solo-watch *Paw Patrol* clips on YouTube and having a parent physically sit next to them and use that very same tablet to play an interactive game. Having a parent and child touch a screen together introduces a whole world of fine motor, social, language, and even gross motor skills.

It's really restrained screen time that's the biggest problem. The observational studies showing increased risk in obesity, social issues, sleep problems all look at sedentary screen use. So even watching those same, terrible YouTube videos while crawling around on the floor and chewing on stuffed animals is a different experience for a toddler than doing so while buckled into a chair.

It's yet another reason that you shouldn't worry so much about time limits. While the AAP does continue to recommend age-based time cutoffs, it also emphasizes that this needs to be part of a larger conversation. Family media planning—creating a framework for how, and how much, screens are used in your household—is a hot topic right now, and for good reason. Embracing the bigger picture of media consumption and setting the stage for healthy screen use throughout childhood and into the teen years, is a crucial parenting task.

Shorter stretches of low-benefit, sedentary screen time seem safer, but I view them as actually more harmful than longer stretches of higher engagement screen-based activity. I'll vote for a rainy afternoon snuggled as a family on the sofa with a full-length movie over a daily, strictly limited thirty-minute session alone with a tablet any day. How both parents and children engage with screens—and each other during screen time—matters more than anything.

5. "Educational" programming is great—but it isn't everything.

Yes, as a pediatrician, it's the law that I support Public Broadcasting. But there's no program that's so educational, such a joy to watch, such a spark to little neurons that it isn't, still, at the end of the day, a TV show. This means that while letting your toddler watch hours of strapped-in *Sesame Street* may seem better than the two of you dancing to a Pinkfong video together, that's not the case. How, how much, and with what framework you consume screens still really matters, even when the content is legitimately educational.

There is still plenty of reason to embrace educational content, and choose higher quality programming whenever you can. As your toddler grows, they are more actively processing the messaging—and subtext—in their media. A PBS Kids show is much more likely to share the values and content you'll want your child to be exposed to (and internalize as something society approves of) than, say, an episode of *Cocomelon* is. These shows also tend to be a bit more interactive, with call-and-response question answering, singing, and even dancing that's certainly better than the trance of watching some other kid open gifts on YouTube.

Higher quality shows are also better for adults! I know that I'm personally less likely to jump on my phone (or run to another room) when an objectively better show is on in the living room—thank you, weirdly hilarious *Odd Squad* for strengthening my daughter's love of absurdist humor and secretly trying to teach her math. Sure, watching this together doesn't count as our "quality time," but cuddling my daughter on the couch is always better, for both of us, than the games-on-my-phone/TV-in-the-background double-screen experience.

6.   *Sometimes, the rules don't apply.*

There will be times when the benefits of using a screen— even a passive one with insipid programming—will be greater than the benefits of stubborn abstinence. When kids are in the hospital, we give them whatever tablets they need to get through poking and prodding, helping them feel safe and comforted as possible. Plane rides are survival of the fittest, and I will keep letting my daughter watch unlimited movies using her adorable toddler headphones for as long as this entertains her (you're welcome, everyone else on our flight). Don't martyr yourself. I promise that the misery from hours of screaming (especially in situations—like long flights—that you can't escape) is much worse than some extra screen time.

It doesn't even have to be an extreme situation. There will absolutely be days when work has been exhausting, life is too stressful, or something is just sapping the last ray of loving, attentive energy and you simply need a break. It's completely okay for YouTube videos to tag in as the nanny to get a few minutes of rest or an extra half hour of "me time."

7. View screen time as negative space.

Don't forget: passive screen time spent watching programming on tablets, phones, and televisions is often replacing time that would have previously been spent on more hands-on interactivity. Think about it: If a six-month-old watches hours of Netflix each day instead of playing with caretakers, doing tummy time, practicing holding and reaching for objects, etc., it makes sense that a delay might develop. That is to say, it may be less about the addition of screens into our lives and more about what they are replacing.

If most of your child's day is spent reading books, playing with caretakers, exploring the world around them, and engaging in other developmentally stimulating activities, there's no need to stress about letting them watch a whole movie (gasp!) one morning so that you can nap for an extra hour.

8. Practice what you preach.

This was (and remains) by far the hardest rule to implement. It's relatively easy to monitor a kid's daily screen exposure, but your own? All parents, like all modern humans, are to varying and increasing degrees slaves to technology. There's nothing like trying to minimize your child's screen time to make you realize just how insanely screen-filled your life is.

Recognizing the role of personal screen use is just as important as any other technology regulation for kids. The time that we spend checking our email or scrolling through social media is time away from our little ones. Sure, we all need some alone time, and if that needs to take the form of a screen binge, that's more than fine. But the key is cognizance. Being aware of this more insidious and passive screen activity is in many ways more important than any other screen regulation. These moments bring all the bad of baby screen exposure—distraction from human interaction, replacing developmental activities—with essentially no real benefit. Other than, as I mention, the very real and important benefit of keeping a technology-dependent parent sane! So while there's no need to ban all adult screen use around infants, just realize that it's another messy part of the equation. Setting some boundaries is helpful, like no phones at the dinner table, even when your kid isn't sitting at the dinner table with you. In the end, modeling reasonable screen behavior from the beginning will help you set the tone for how you want your family to interface with technology as your little one grows.

9. Video chat gets a free pass—at least until we invent holograms (or teleportation).

The AAP is completely okay with FaceTime and other video chatting, and so am I. Studies show that the social and emotional benefits of staying connected with families not only neutralize the "risks" of screen exposure but also likely outweigh them. How could anyone deny the importance to the entire family of showing grandparents, friends, families how your infant is doing and enhancing these bonds over geographical distances? As I'm sure no one needs reminding, the pandemic made spending time physically together in the same room harder than ever. My toddler and I FaceTimed friends and family for hours each day that we were stuck in strict quarantine during the spring 2020 New York covid surge. There was no doubt in my mind that the benefit of virtual interaction with other children was enormous compared to any potential risk.

10. Set yourself up for success.

Strict time limits may be so 2016, but it's okay to have some restrictions. Creating healthy boundaries and even some ground rules is a good way to make sure you don't let the passive onslaught of screens take over your baby's life. This might be some simple interior design—like facing the TV away from your dining area and committing to sit-down mealtimes, even when your child isn't around.

I like to view the issue of screen time as less of a daily one and more week-to-week. If we go three days with no TV, then indulge in a rainy-day movie marathon, I don't sweat it. But if our work and childcare situations are relatively stable, and it's been a few days in a row of more than an hour with Netflix as the nanny, I make a mental note to try to make some scheduling changes for the rest of the week.

THE BOTTOM LINE

5 out of 5 Pediatrician Parents Agree

1. Some screen exposure is inevitable, even for toddlers. It's easier to form a healthy relationship with screens if you embrace their ubiquity. It's better to pivot from abstinence toward a more deliberate, flexible approach.

2. When it comes to screen time for little kids, less is usually more. Daily limits from the AAP can be a good starting point but are hard to stick to for many, many families. If strict cutoffs aren't working, try to focus instead on weekly averages and patterns of screen use.

3. Not all screens are created equal, and how screens are used really matters! For example, there is a world of difference between sedentary, passive, and especially *restrained* solo video watching and an interactive game or family movie night.

4. Every parenting decision is a balance of risk and benefit for your individual situation, and screens are no exception. You will consider your unique circumstances, personal privilege, life's realities, and what works for your family when deciding on how and how much screens are used. Each decision is also a moment in time, and there will be situations where exceeding even the limits you've deliberately set will have more benefit than harm.

5. Educational programs still aren't everything. A marathon of *Sesame Street* and *NOVA* documentaries can't replace the developmental benefit of free play and in-person interaction. However, as your toddler grows, more actively processes messages and subtext from media, and consumes more of it, paying more attention to the quality of programming makes sense.

6. The hardest part of screen time moderation is focusing on your *own* consumption. It's also the most important. Doubling down on your own relationship with your screen—both the amount of time you spend and if/how it's altering your engagement with the world—will benefit your child more than anything.

7. Excessive screen time is harmful in large part because it acts as "negative space," often replacing other developmentally beneficial activities. All the more reason not to jump to guilt or worry when you consciously choose screen use as part of a parenting style that's filled with interaction and play.

Acknowledgments

"**S**o, when's your book coming out?"

What started as a sort of inside joke as I answered an increasing number of questions from new-parent friends (and friends of friends, and friends of friends of friends) led to an over-five-year-long process of successfully publishing *two* books. It's still surreal. And I absolutely could not have done any of it without the incredible people who supported me at every step.

Thank you to Stuart Reid for not only being the first to suggest that writing a book was something I should seriously pursue, but for then showing me exactly how to make that dream possible. Thank you to Sara Manning Peskin, the inspiring physician-mom and author and friend who also edited my attempt at a proposal and helped me find my agents.

To my agents Justin Brouckaert and Todd Shuster, I'm still amazed that you knew that my passion for realistic, safe parenting advice could turn into these powerhouse books. Thank you for pushing me every step of the way and allowing me to find this singular voice as a parenting author. Justin, I still can't get over just how many back-and-forth edits you patiently went through with my proposal, and will always be grateful for the time you took to help me shape my writing for the better.

Thank you to everyone at Kensington for believing in these books unconditionally and integrally, often more than I even believed in them myself. To Denise Silvestro, my phenomenal editor, who helped this first-time author wade through the exciting (and sometimes overwhelming) process of actually writing my books. To Ann Pryor, who has spent so much effort in publicizing my books and is the reason they will reach the audience that needs them most.

These books come from the deepest parts of my being. They stem from my true sense of self, a feeling of worth and love that I maintain through my family and friends. And I'm so lucky to be loved and supported by so many. I can only "parent like a pediatrician" because of the parenting I have myself been fortunate enough to receive. To my parents, who showed me from the very beginning that unconditional love for a child is simply an expectation. To my mom, a badass doctor-mom herself who made raising four children look easy. There has never been a more devoted mother and I continue to use your parenting as a source of inspiration. To my dad, who actively loved and supported his children before society routinely expected this of fathers.

Thank you to each and every member of my large, warm, messy, and wonderful family, who continue to support me in all that I do. To my three incredible brothers, who continue to outshine me so spectacularly that I am filled with far more pride than jealousy. To my aunts, uncles, cousins, grandparents, nieces, nephews: Growing up alongside so many of you is what helped me become the person I am today. Thank you for always being there for me, and for bringing new and wonderful people into our family. Nana and Poppop, I hope it's always been clear how much of who I am has been shaped by you, and how grateful I am. Nana, your legacy shines through the endless accomplishments of the family you created. You were the mother of mothers, our matriarch, and my biggest cheerleader. I miss you every day, and I know you would have loved these books.

To my amazing friends, who continue to inspire and encourage me daily. Hilary Haimes, Katelyn O'Connor, Susanna O'Kula, the incredible doctors and original support team: I am so grateful to have found you and to still have you in my life. Katharine Magliocco, to say I would be lost without you remains the world's greatest understatement. Thank you for being my number one fan, unpaid brand manager, life coach, and true friend. Emily Rassel, my one-time co-parent and all-time pediatrician-mom idol. Phoebe Danziger, my mind-twin who started me on this writing journey way back when, continues to inspire and intimidate me in the best of ways. To the local MM crew—Amy, Claire, Paul, Stuart, and the wee ones—that has become my lifeline and keeps me sane, thank you for being here for me every day.

Thank you to the experts who so graciously shared their wisdom with me and helped me provide evidence-based guidance in these books. Melissa Glassman, Ellie Erickson,

Cristina Fernandez, Rebecca Schrag Hershberg, and countless other brilliant colleagues and role models showed me how doctor-moms can speak up and make a difference.

Like so many parents, I wouldn't be able to do anything without the incredible efforts of childcare workers. Thank you to the nannies and babysitters who have helped me raise my daughters to be the wonderful people they are. I couldn't have accomplished any of this without knowing they were safe in your care.

I share my own mental and physical health struggles throughout this book so others will feel empowered to get the help they need. Thank you to my own health-care team. To my amazing OB physicians, without whom I literally wouldn't be alive. Dr. Pasque, I still look to you as a model for my work both as a physician and as a supporter of parents. To my own psychiatrist and therapist, thank you for getting me through everything.

And above all, this book is dedicated to the loves of my life. To my husband, thank you for being you. You are the best partner I could ever have hoped for, and a greater father than I ever could have imagined existed. And to my daughters, whom I love more than words can ever express: Everything I do is to make the world a better place for both of you. You are my light, my joy, my proudest accomplishments. The greatest privilege and pleasure in my life is being able to call myself your mommy.

Index

INDEX

Index

control, toddlers' lack of, 263
control of child's eating, 156–57, 160
conversations on hard topics, 255–67
cortisol, 104–105, 108
coughing, 185, 198, 199, 204, 205
COVID-19, 222–23, 224–27. *See also*
pandemic parenting
cow's milk, 137, 138, 147
CPR, 235
crib, transition from, 186–87, 188
critical thinking, 38
curiosity. *See* inquisitiveness

dairy, 137
data-driven parenting, 6, 8, 226
daycare, 275, 278
    separation anxiety, 96, 106–107,
        108–109
    tantrum strategies, 54
    toilet-training requirement, 72, 86
    turn-taking symbols, 26
death, talking to toddler about, 255, 258,
    259–60
decision-making by toddlers, 16, 17
deep breathing, 30, 63, 67
DEET, 247–48
deficiency, nutritional, 152
dehydration, 200, 202
dental devices to stop thumb-sucking,
    121, 131
development of toddlers, 269–78. *See*
    also milestones
    crib, transition from, 186–87
    emotional dysregulation, 15–18
    habits, 115–32
    infant to toddler, 97–99
    screen exposure effects, 284–85, 287
    separation anxiety, 95–114
    solid food, 145
    toilet training, necessary or not,
        72–74, 83–84
developmentally appropriate
    conversations, 259, 262, 266
deviation, 44–45
diapers, dehydration check, 200
diarrhea, 198, 200, 222

diet. *See* nutrition
diphtheria, 220
direct-to-parent marketing, 146
discipline, replacing traditional types, 32
diversity, talking to toddler about, 258
DNA antigens, 223
dolls
    modeling desired behaviors with,
        78, 88
    pediatrician visit preparation, 195
drowning, 243, 252
dysregulation, emotional, 13–39, 60,
    67, 70

early-elimination toilet training method,
    79–81
eating
    exploratory behavior, 19, 151, 154
    picky eating, 149–61
    reinforcement strategy, 89–90
    solid food, transition to, 135–48
eczema, 251
education, toddler, 277, 278
educational television, 288, 293
effortful control, 16
ehrlichiosis, 245
elbow guards, 121–22, 125–26, 131
emergencies, medical, 197–98, 199, 201,
    204
emotional intelligence, 59
emotional problem-solving, 65
emotional regulation, 113
emotional separation, parent from child,
    110–11
emotions
    anger management, 63
    development, 13–18
    dysregulation, 13–39
    emotional tools, 21–23
    emotions, parental anxiety, 193
    feelings vs. behavior, 62
    parents' responses, 56–57
    self-regulation, 110–11
    separation anxiety, 96–97, 113
    tantrums, 57–58, 60, 66–68
    transitions, 261

301

INDEX